WHAT ABOUT THE FAMILY?

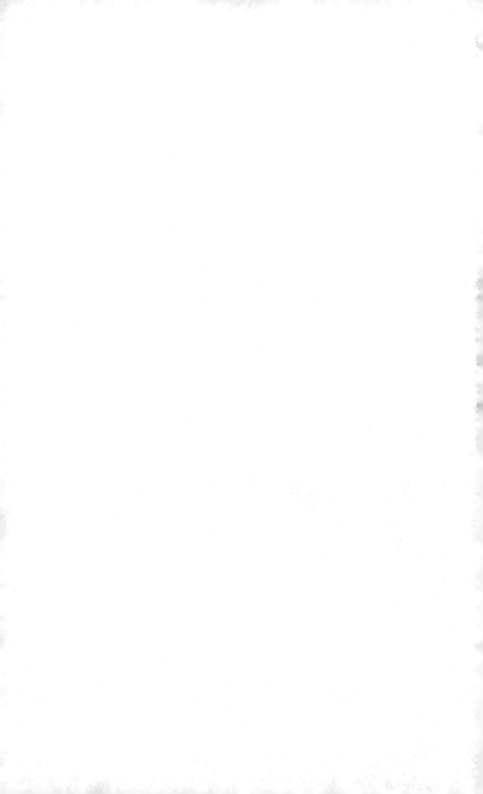

WHAT ABOUT THE FAMILY?

Practices of Responsibility in Care

Edited by Marian A. Verkerk

Hilde Lindemann

AND

Janice McLaughlin

OXFORD
UNIVERSITY PRESS

OXFORD
UNIVERSITY PRESS

Oxford University Press is a department of the University of Oxford. It furthers
the University's objective of excellence in research, scholarship, and education
by publishing worldwide. Oxford is a registered trade mark of Oxford University
Press in the UK and certain other countries.

Published in the United States of America by Oxford University Press
198 Madison Avenue, New York, NY 10016, United States of America.

Library of Congress Cataloging-in-Publication Data
Names: Verkerk, Marian, editor.
Title: What about the family? : practices of responsibility in care /
edited by Marian A. Verkerk, Hilde Lindemann, and Janice McLaughlin.
Description: New York, NY : Oxford University Press, [2019] |
Includes bibliographical references and index.
Identifiers: LCCN 2018053832 (print) | LCCN 2018061615 (ebook) |
ISBN 9780190624897 (Online content) | ISBN 9780190624903 (updf) |
ISBN 9780190624910 (epub) | ISBN 9780190624880 (cloth : alk. paper)
Subjects: LCSH: Families--Health and hygiene. | Responsibility. |
Bioethics. Classification: LCC RA418.5.F3 (ebook) |
LCC RA418.5.F3 W43 2019 (print) | DDC 613—dc23
LC record available at https://lccn.loc.gov/2018053832

1 3 5 7 9 8 6 4 2

Printed by Sheridan Books, Inc., United States of America

CONTENTS

Contributors   *ix*

Introduction   1
Janice McLaughlin, Hilde Lindemann,
and Marian A. Verkerk

1. Why Families Matter   16
Hilde Lindemann

Case Study: Lesbian Parents' Search for the "Right
    Way" to Disclose Donor Conception
    to Their Children   36
Veerle Provoost

2. Recognizing Family   47
Janice McLaughlin

Case Study: The Family Imperative in Genetic Testing   70
Lorraine Cowley

Case Study: What Counts as a Family—And Who Is
    to Decide?   80
Margareta Hydén

3. Negotiating Responsibilities   89
Marian A. Verkerk

Case Study: Paternal Responsibility for Children
    and Pediatric Hospital Policies in Romania   100
Daniela Cutaş and Anca Gheauş

Case Study: Family Caregiving as a Problematic
    Category   109
Jacqueline Chin

4. Healthcare Decisions   118
Ulrik Kihlbom and Christian Munthe

Case Study: Family Centeredness as Resource and
    Complication in Outpatient Care with Weak
    Adherence, Using Adolescent Diabetes Care as a
    Case in Point   137
Anders Herlitz and Christian Munthe

Case Study: Annie's Problem   147
Jackie Leach Scully

5. Justice, Intimacy, and Autonomy   155
Jamie Lindemann Nelson and Simon Woods

Case Study: Young Caregivers   176
Gideon Calder

Case Study: Autism, Family Life, and
  Epistemic Injustice   183
  Richard Ashcroft

Index   189

CONTRIBUTORS

Richard Ashcroft is Professor of Bioethics in the School of Law at Queen Mary University of London. He is the author of more than 200 academic publications in the field of bioethics, with particular interests in research ethics and public health ethics.

Gideon Calder is Director of the Social Policy Programme at Swansea University, working primarily on social justice and applied ethics. He is author or co-editor of ten books, most recently *The Routledge Handbook of the Philosophy of Childhood and Children*, and co-edits the journal *Ethics & Social Welfare*. His current research focuses on co-production, and what equality means for children.

Jacqueline Chin is Associate Professor at the Centre for Biomedical Ethics (CBmE), Yong Loo Lin School of Medicine, National University of Singapore. Her research addresses national and globally relevant capacity building in biomedical ethics, including *What Doctors Say About Care of the Dying*, a study of doctors' perspectives on end-of-life decisions (2010–2011); *Making Difficult Decisions with Patients and Families* (2014), volume 1 of an online casebook (www.bioethicscasebook.sg) featured in a collection of papers on Bioethics Education 2015 by the US Presidential Commission for the Study of Bioethical Issues; and volume 2, *Caring for Older People in an Ageing Society* (2017), which engages with ethical challenges of eldercare in community care settings.

Lorraine Cowley is Principal Genetic Counsellor at the Institute of Genomic Medicine in Newcastle, United Kingdom. Her background is in cancer nursing since 1990 and cancer genetic counselling since 1997. She has a PhD in Sociology from Newcastle University where she was based in PEALS (Policy Ethics and Life Sciences) and funded by Cancer Research UK and Wellcome Trust. Her research interests are in how mainstreaming genetic testing influences moral understandings of genetic testing for disease susceptibility genes.

Daniela Cutaş is Associate Professor in Practical Philosophy at Umeå University and the University of Gothenburg. She is a co-editor of the volumes *Families: Beyond the Nuclear Ideal* (2012) and *Parental Responsibility in the Context of Neuroscience and Genetics* (2017).

Anca Gheauş is a Ramon y Cajal Fellow / Researcher at the Law Department at Universitat Pompeu Fabra (Barcelona). She also works as a member of the Family Justice project, funded by the European Research Council Consolidator Grants program. Before that she had research positions at the University College Dublin, Erasmus University Rotterdam, University of Sheffield and University of Umea. Her main work is on theories of distributive justice, with a particular focus on the family and gender justice.

Anders Herlitz is an expert on distributive ethics and population-level bioethics and has published widely in these areas. Recent articles by Herlitz have appeared in *Social Science and Medicine, Health Communications, Journal of Medical Ethics,* and other outlets. He is currently Marie Curie Fellow at the Department of Global Health and Population at Harvard University, and Researcher in Philosophy at the University of Gothenburg.

Margareta Hydén is Emerita Professor in Social Work at Linköping University, Sweden, and a guest professor in criminology at Stockholm University, Sweden. Her major area of research concerns interpersonal violence. She has also studied agency in women's narratives of leaving abusive relationships and has developed narrative approaches for the study of sensitive topics. Professor Hydén is currently conducting research on the victims' and perpetrators' social networks' responses to violence.

Ulrik Kihlbom is Associate Professor and Senior Lecturer in Medical Ethics at the Centre for Research Ethics & Bioethics, Uppsala University. He has long been responsible for the course in Medical Ethics and Medical Law at the Uppsala University Medical School. His main research interests are methodology of bioethics, ethical particularism, patient autonomy, and clinical decision making.

Hilde Lindemann is Emerita Professor of Philosophy at Michigan State University. A Fellow of the Hastings Center and a past president of the American Society for Bioethics and Humanities, her ongoing research interests are in feminist bioethics, feminist ethics, the ethics of families, and the social construction of persons and their identities. She is author or co-editor of eight books, including, with James Lindemann Nelson, *The Patient in the Family*. Her most recent book is *Holding and Letting Go: The Social Practice of Personal Identities*.

Janice McLaughlin is a sociologist who studies various aspects of childhood disability and family life. In a number of projects and publications, she has explored the experiences of disabled children and their families within health and social care. Her most recent book is *Disabled Childhoods: Monitoring Difference and Emerging Identities.*

Christian Munthe is Professor of Practical Philosophy at the Department of Philosophy, Linguistics and Theory of Science at the University of Gothenburg in Sweden. Focusing on ethics and value issues in the intersection of health, science and technology, the environment, and society, his recent areas of research include the ethics of person centeredness and shared decision making in healthcare and social work.

Jamie Lindemann Nelson is Professor of Philosophy at Michigan State University, a Fellow of the Hastings Center, and a co-editor of the *International Journal of Feminist Approaches to Bioethics.* She is the co-author (with Hilde Lindemann) of *The Patient in the Family* and of *Alzheimer's: Answers to Hard Questions for Families,* as well as the author of some hundred articles in bioethics.

Veerle Provoost is Professor of Empirical Research in Moral Science and Ethics, and a member of BIG (Bioethics Institute Ghent) at Ghent University in Belgium. She is a philosopher and social health scientist with research interests in family members' and lay people's moral decision-making. Over the past seven years, she coordinated an interdisciplinary team of researchers who studied genetic and social parenthood in the context of donor conception.

Jackie Leach Scully is Professor of Social Ethics and Bioethics, and Executive Director of PEALS (Policy, Ethics and Life Sciences Research Centre) at Newcastle University in the United Kingdom. She is a Fellow of the Academy of Arts and Sciences. Originally a molecular biologist, she has been active in bioethics for nearly twenty years, with particular research interests in feminist bioethics, disability bioethics, new genetic and reproductive technologies, and the moral understandings of non-professional publics, including patients.

Marian A. Verkerk is Full Professor of Ethics of Care at the University Medical Centre Groningen and the University of Groningen. She was project leader of the Network of Family Ethics from 2011 to 2017. She is the author of more than 150 academic (national and international) publications in the field of bioethics, with particular interests in care ethics and palliative care. Among other organizations, she has been a member of the Health Council of the Netherlands (2004–2016), a member of the Review Committee on Euthanasia (1999–2012), and Chair of the Committee on Palliative Sedation of the Royal Medical Association of the Netherlands. She is currently project leader on Patient Participation at the University Medical Centre Groningen.

Simon Woods is Reader in Bioethics and Deputy Director of the Policy Ethics and Life Sciences Research Institute at Newcastle University UK. He is a philosopher and former oncology nurse who works on the social and ethical issues within the life sciences and health care. His published work engages with topics including end-of-life ethics, rare disease genomics, and research ethics.

Introduction

JANICE MCLAUGHLIN, HILDE LINDEMANN,
AND MARIAN A. VERKERK

In 2010, the Dutch bioethicist Marian Verkerk created the Consortium on the Ethics of Families in Health and Social Care. The consortium emerged out of the long-term research contributions of Verkerk, Lindemann, and Nelson (Lindemann et al. 2008; Nelson and Lindemann Nelson 1995) to philosophically evaluating the significance of family to healthcare practices. Their different work has over the years asked a key justice question: Is it fair for health and social care professionals to assume that when people are ill or need extra care that this can and indeed should be supplied by family?

Their work was an important catalyst to a range of bioethics researchers taking up the question over the last two decades. There is now an ongoing and important debate about the nature and quality of familial obligations and rights in healthcare contexts. Researchers have explored whether shared responsibilities operate between a family and the individuals within it simply as a result of being a family unit, without contestation, conflict, or inequality (Hardwig 1990; Ho 2008). For example, bioethicists are now asking if it is reasonable to assume that family members will support others in the family, in ways that will sustain them, both during periods of crisis and across a life in need of care (Cassidy 2013; Levine 2000). Another area of consideration is whether patients, while sustained and supported by families who care for them, should still be thought of as individuals by the health and social care professionals who treat them—in other words, that families' needs and viewpoints on what the person needs should be seen as outside the concern of the practitioner (Brighouse and Swift 2014; Kinjo and Morioka 2011).

The consortium was created to bring new light to these debates by moving it forward in several key ways. The first was to expand to issues of social care as well as healthcare, given their close interaction. For example, decisions about when someone should leave the hospital are often led by considerations of whether social services are in place to support the person back in the community. The second key way was to draw into the debate other disciplinary perspectives to introduce different ideas on what is involved in interrogating the relationship between families and health and social care. This comes from recognition that within areas such as anthropology, sociology, nursing, literary studies, theology, and disability studies, questions about familial responsibility for care have been a longstanding point of contention. Drawing from these perspectives helps us to understand more fully individuals within the relations of intimacy that support them as human beings, influence their decision making, and generate their responsibilities to others and others' to them. Third, drawing in these different perspectives has enabled greater questioning of what it is we speak of when we speak of family.

In particular, we have drawn on anthropological work that explores how kinship connections form in different societies and cultures (Carsten 2000; Strathern 1992)—for example, how cultural values validate the different kinship connections people live within and make moral judgements about (Franklin and McKinnon

2001); historical research studying the relationship between social change and the formation of familial boundaries—for example, changes from extended family living to nuclear family households (Gillis 1996); and sociological work on family, whether this be feminist research on the division of labor in families (Finch and Mason 1993) or the more recent interest in how people make kinship ties that are not centered on heterosexuality and reproduction (Morgan 1996; Weeks et al. 2001).

Consortium members came from the UK, Sweden, Singapore, Germany, the Netherlands, and the US to discuss what counts as a family, why families matter, and how they operate. The series of meetings resulted in a paper, "Where Families and Health Care Meet," published in the *Journal of Medical Ethics* (Verkerk et al. 2015). In 2014 Verkerk received a grant from the Netherlands Organization of Scientific Research to continue the work of the consortium, and the idea for this edited collection was born. Co-funding support was also provided by Michigan State University, Newcastle University, Groningen University, Lübeck University, Gothenburg University, Uppsala University, and Linköping University.

The book is one result of the many productive cross-disciplinary discussions that have taken place. The conversations aim to understand better the interrelationships between people receiving health and social care, those intimate to them, and the range of practitioners they may encounter in their lives. The book also gives a strong priority to engaging with the implications for policy and practice. Themes explored have included, among others, how familial-type relationships inform people's approach to living with illness or disability, the choices they make around treatment options, and the influence of broader social and cultural values on the responsibilities they enact with others and expect enacted for them. Two key themes unite the varied contributions of our different chapter authors: (1) questions of responsibility and (2) understandings of narrative. In the next two sections we will discuss these two themes, before then describing the approach of the book and its structure.

I. CARE RESPONSIBILITIES

There are a number of reasons why the collection centers on the question of responsibility. First, significant advances in contemporary medicine have put moral and practical pressure on families and health and social care providers alike. Such advances are enabling people to live longer, sometimes well, sometimes not, with a range of health conditions and disabilities. This means that medical innovation is generating extended and varied forms of care needs, which are distributed among a range of actors. This produces complex questions of with whom and for what do responsibilities lie. More is being asked of families, in terms of providing care and also being party to the complex decisions faced by family members receiving complex treatment. Health and social care practitioners are aware that familial relationships are affected by and are a background for what they provide, and so must be drawn upon when navigating pathways of care. What is not always clear, however, is how to do that in the context of treating people who should be enabled to make their own decisions, in their own best interests.

Second, long-term social changes, played out differently in different global and local contexts, are affecting the formations of family ties, in particular the availability of family members to take on different responsibilities and the competing demands on family to provide care (Beck 1997). Familial and intimate relationships need consideration because they are not static, self-evident entities (Beck and Beck-Gernsheim 2002). Instead there have been long-term, significant changes in how people "do" family in many societies, so it is important to be wary of assumptions about who is family, who are its primary caregivers, and where boundaries of responsibility lie. For example, greater gender equality and women's presence in the world of work make it less sustainable to see women as the primary caregivers within their close and extended families, a change affecting not just the Global North but also the emerging capitalist economies of much of Asia (Fan 2007; Okin 1989; Walby 1997). At the same time the demographic trend, supported by medicine, that people are living longer can mean that women can find themselves at the center of intergenerational care needs, while also in paid employment (Conlon et al. 2014).

Third, greater care also has to be taken with how intimate relationships that matter are identified and are attended to in questions regarding responsibility. For example, there is increased recognition that people live within ties of intimacy and care in many different ways: same-sex families, "blended" families made up of offspring from multiple relationships, people articulating their close friendships as being their "chosen" familial setting, and people living apart but together (Jamieson 1998). Such relationship forms are not necessarily new but are now given greater legal and cultural recognition in many global contexts. In such contexts questions of who has or should have responsibility are tied also to how intimate ties are recognized and valued in different health and social care settings.

A final reason for a focus on responsibility is that, in much of the Global North at least, we have seen retrenchment of provision within health and social care and a turn toward private responsibility to look after oneself both financially and in avoiding ill health (Lupton 1995; Rose 2006). Governments are actively appealing to families to look after their own to fill the care gap of an aging society. However, it is not so obvious who "our own" are and what duty we owe them, particularly if we also consider the responsibilities of the state to provide for its citizens and to protect against inequality and injustice.

All of these factors (and others) are producing intersecting pressure points for people who need health and social care support, providers, and expected caregivers. In this collection, by examining how these responsibilities are assumed and assigned, shared and deflected, the different contributions demonstrate the practical importance of a distinctive ethics of families. They also indicate the importance of retaining a critical questioning of what and whom is being drawn into ethical consideration when speaking of "family." This is why we speak of *ethics of family* rather than *family ethics*.

II. NARRATIVE

Each contributor to the collection shares an interest in narrative aspects of family and intimate relationships, medical decision making, and moral life. Narratives, in varied ways, are seen as part of what sustain people in relationships, inform understandings of responsibility, and allow decisions to make sense to those involved (Lindemann 2014). In stories people tell about who they are and who they think of as family, they represent what matters to them while also being informed by the stories available and recognizable within their social worlds (Finch 2007; McCarthy et al. 2000). Narratives (the shape or style a story takes) are not only personal but social and cultural. This affects what kinds of stories can be told and recognized by others (Lawler 2008). This point also means that the contributors share a commitment to questions about inequality and justice. What stories are possible are influenced by existing social hierarchies that make judgments about acceptable ways of life (Poletta et al. 2011; Riessman 1993). For example, the dominance of stories of families as being essentially heteronormative has precluded the recognition of same-sex intimacies as being of equal value to opposite-sex intimacies (Taylor 2009). This has had significant implications in health and social care when, for example, a same-sex partner has not been recognized as next of kin and has been excluded from being part of decisions about someone's care. The power of this narrative is lessening with the increasing legal recognition of same-sex marriage, although it still excludes those who object to marriage being required to be recognized as next of kin (Richardson 2005).

III. THE COLLECTION'S CENTRAL QUESTION AND APPROACHES

If families, however people conceive of them, are responsible for providing the care needed to sustain family members who are receiving health or social care, who is it that bears this responsibility, on what basis do they bear it, and what is the nature of the responsibility?

Across the collection, not all contributors approach this question or indeed answer it in the same way. This we see as a virtue of bringing together the different disciplinary perspectives and bodies of research in the consortium. There are differences among authors on whether family relations, of whatever form, have within them certain qualities that generate specific responsibilities. Nor do all contributors speak in a single voice about what the implications are of recognizing that family relationships can be deeply problematic; they can be abusive, people can be estranged, yet they can still articulate a sense of obligation in such contexts. What to do about and with such obligations in contexts of dysfunction remains a vital and important area of debate.

Contributors do agree on some important key points. There is a strong emphasis given to families as encompassing varied social and intimate relationships, which can include intergenerational ties, but not necessarily so. It is the relationships, often but not always called family, which people frame as deeply meaningful to them in their intimate lives that are the collection's focus. The bioethics literature is apt to dwell on the sexy stuff: novel technologies, questions of life and death, and dramatic moral dilemmas that arise infrequently. These, to be sure, are important. However, many of the researchers brought together here focus instead on the everyday tensions around how people live in and form family relationships, how they experience and care for long-term and chronic illness, and how day-to-day decisions and practices are also sites of moral judgment.

All the contributors are researchers actively working on understanding the medical and social perplexities that lie behind the creation of the collection. An additional benefit of drawing bioethics into consideration with other disciplinary perspectives on family is that it enables the inclusion of empirical research into the debate (Haimes 2002). The contributors examine what a range of actors do when faced with dilemmas. Rich work across multiple contexts explores why and how people live with each other, the care responsibilities they enact, and the decisions they make. The end product could be summarized as a form of "naturalized moral epistemology" in bioethics (Lindemann et al. 2008). Each contributor takes moral knowledge to be found only here and now, in real time. We share a belief that idealized moral theories could work properly only in the ideal societies imagined to be in strict compliance with them, not in the actual world where there is a plurality of moral traditions and norms are routinely violated. Morality does not set controls on how we are to respond to the human condition in an ideal world of order and plenty, but in our own world—a world where people are flawed, where human connection is both important and difficult to maintain, and where the value of cooperation and trust is inseparable from the disvalue of vulnerability and competition (Baier 1985, 218). The problems with an idealized moral epistemology are twofold: not only does an idealized approach to justification fail precisely where moral norms cannot be defended in actual practice, but ideal theory's assumptions leave us with guidance that is either too vague to be useful in hard cases or so precisely specific that we would constantly have to wonder about legitimate exceptions. For those reasons, the contributors here work across both empirically and theoretically based research so that they can move back and forth between what happens in different social realities and normative questions about morality, social justice, and the good life.

Ultimately, what the contributors share is an intent to fully engage with relationships characterized by ongoing intimacy and partiality among people who are not interchangeable. All are very much centered on the practices of responsibility arising from these relationships. There is, of course, a great deal more work to do than brought together here, and we call upon future researchers in these areas to carry this work forward. For one thing, the book does not say very much here about how love operates in families or what love is. More needs to be said about families' role in caring for disabled or elderly members, or for disabled and elderly members' role in caring for those who care for them. Finally, much more work is needed to consider the roles society plays or ought to play in the interactions between families and health and social care. All the same, the questions asked here and the conclusions reached seem worth consideration, so we do hope others will take up where the collection ends.

IV. STRUCTURE

Each chapter of the collection works through a set of questions that provide a framework for understanding the problematic behind the book and the broader debates it is part of: why families matter, what counts as family, how families track responsibilities, how treatment decisions ought to work in families, and what justice requires of families. Each chapter ends with two case studies or commentaries (except Chapter 1, which has one case study), which either illustrate some point the chapter is making or test the theoretical resources the chapter offers. The case study authors, who come from a range of disciplinary backgrounds and international contexts, examine specific situations where families and health and social care interact. Some case studies are fictional while others come from empirical research, enabling the reader to see that we can build up from thinking about how things occur in practice as well as draw down from more abstract, theoretical concepts. The idea is to achieve equilibrium: the empirical data put pressure on the theorizing, while the theories allow the data to be interpreted.

Chapter 1.

Hilde Lindemann is a philosopher who has spent her career examining the significance of family to people's sense of self and their experiences of healthcare. In this chapter she makes a case for families' being of consequence. She does so by arguing that families, of varied form and size and shape, and across our lifetime, enable us to flourish. Therefore, they are central to our experiences of illness and disability and the decisions this may generate for us. In the case study in Chapter 1, Veerle Provoost draws from empirical research undertaken with lesbian couples who have used donor conception services in Belgium to trace how existing norms of family life influence the way they interacted with the services and made sense of the choices they made.

Chapter 2.

Janice McLaughlin is a sociologist whose empirical and theoretical work includes examinations of family life in contexts such as childhood disability. Her chapter looks at the influence of social and cultural processes in how families are recognized both as family and "the right kind" of family. Questions of power and inequality are identified as central to dynamics of recognition. In the first case study in Chapter 2, Lorraine Cowley, a genetics counselor, examines how members of an extended family network in Northern England with a shared history of genetic risk for cancer made choices about whether to have a genetic test, influenced by their social understandings of who their family was and what responsibilities came with that. In the second case study in Chapter 2, Margareta Hydén, a clinical psychologist, highlights how understandings of what a "real" family is can get in the way of responding to a child in need. She does this through her account of interactions with one young person in a Swedish research project who made new forms of familial connection with others after difficult struggles with her original kin.

Chapter 3.

Marian Verkerk is a philosopher who examines how moral stances in a range of health and social care contexts emerge and are lived in contexts of social vulnerability and ambiguity. In this chapter she looks at some of the ethical implications being created by the ways in which families are increasingly required to step in to take responsibility for people in need. Such requirements are ethically complex because someone may feel an obligation to act even though this may be unjust due to past family histories of harm and abuse. In the first case study in Chapter 3, Daniela Cutaş and Anca Gheauş, feminist philosophers, make use of current legal and policy debates in Romania over the rights of fathers to be recognized as important caregivers in hospital settings to show that gendered family norms can problematically shape who is allowed to care for an ill child. Jacqueline Chin, a bioethicist, then works with a hypothetical case study to examine complex social and intimate interactions of care between paid and family caregivers and an elderly woman in need of intensive daily care in Singapore.

Chapter 4.

Ulrik Kihlbom and Christian Munthe are philosophers interested in how values and moral beliefs, including ideas of what a good life and a good family are, influence people's interactions with health and social care. In this chapter, in the context of the increased call for patients to be involved in shared decision making, the focus is on how such shared decision making can involve family members as well. Their argument is that while family can and should become part of shared decision-making dynamics, care needs to be taken over how this is done, in particular what assumptions are made about who are the relevant family members to include. In the first case study in Chapter 4, Anders Herlitz and Christian Munthe, both philosophers, draw from their Swedish research on young people's compliance with diabetes treatment to show ways in which family members can (and should not) be brought into patient-led care. In the second case study, Jackie Leach Scully, a feminist bioethicist, lays out the case of a sister in the UK considering whether to participate in a pool of shared donation in order to help her brother, for whom she is not a match. She examines how donating to someone else to in the end help the brother is lived as a different experience to donating directly.

Chapter 5.

Jamie Lindemann Nelson and Simon Woods are philosophers who work across political theory and bioethics to critically evaluate the fairness of what happens to individuals in spaces of complex health and social care interaction. In this final substantial chapter they take questions of family responsibility into the realm of theorizing on justice. They work with a range of approaches to justice to consider the dilemmas emerging over the fairness of what is being asked of family members in contexts of resource scarcity and significant economic inequality. In the first case study in Chapter 4, Gideon Calder, a social and political theorist, lays out a hypothetical story of a young girl in the UK drawn into significant caring responsibilities for her sibling and mother, exploring whether it is just and fair for her to have such responsibilities, while acknowledging the value the young girl herself sees in the role she plays and the person she has become. In the second case study, Richard Ashcroft, a philosopher, explores the important social and resource challenges children with autism and their families face in receiving appropriate care and support from the healthcare system in the UK. He reflects on his own experiences as the father of an autistic son and asks whether it is just to speak for his son.

ACKNOWLEDGMENTS

The book is also the result of extensive discussions we had during our workshops over three years. Accordingly, we want to thank Christopher Rehman-Sutter, Christina Schues, and Kristin Zeiler for their very valuable contributions. We also want to thank John Hardwig, whose seminal 1990 paper in the *Hastings Center Report* began the discussion in bioethics of families. The title of our collection pays homage to that paper.

REFERENCES

Baier, Annette. 1985. "Theory and Reflective Practices." In *Postures of the Mind: Essays on Mind and Morals*, 207–27. Minneapolis: University of Minnesota Press.

Beck, Ulrich. 1997. "Democratization of the Family." *Childhood* 4: 151–168.

Beck, Ulrich, and Elizabeth Beck-Gernsheim. 2002. *Individualization: Institutionaliz ed Individualism and Its Social and Political Consequences.* Chichester, UK: Wiley.

Brighouse, Harry, and Adam Swift. 2014. *Family Values: The Ethics of Parent–Child Relationships.* Princeton, NJ: Princeton University Press.

Carsten, Janet. 2000. *Cultures of Relatedness.* Cambridge, UK: Cambridge University Press.

Cassidy, Lisa. 2013. "Thoughts on the Bioethics of Estranged Biological Kin." *Hypatia: A Journal of Feminist Philosophy* 28: 32–48.

Conlon, Catherine, Virpi Timonen, Gemma Carney, and Thomas Scharf. 2014. "Women (Re) Negotiating Care Across Family Generations: Intersections of Gender and Socioeconomic Status." *Gender & Society* 28: 729–51.

Fan, Ruiping. 2007. "Which Care? Whose Responsibility? And Why Family? A Confucian Account of Long-Term Care for the Elderly." *Journal of Medicine and Philosophy: A Forum for Bioethics and Philosophy* 32: 495–517.

Finch, Janet. 2007. "Displaying Families." *Sociology* 41: 65–81.

Finch, Janet, and Jennifer Mason. 1993. *Negotiating Family Responsibilities.* London: Routledge.

Franklin, Sarah, and Susan McKinnon. 2001. "Relative Values: Reconfiguring Kinship Studies." In *Relative Values: Reconfiguring Kinship Studies,* ed. Sarah Franklin and Susan McKinnon, eds., 1–28. Durham, NC: Duke University Press.

Gillis, John R. 1996. *A World of Their Own Making.* Boston, MA: Harvard University Press.

Haimes, Erica. 2002. "What Can the Social Sciences Contribute to the Study of Ethics? Theoretical, Empirical and Substantive Considerations." *Bioethics* 16: 89–113.

Hardwig, John. 1990. "What About the Family?" *Hastings Center Report* 20(2): 5–10.

Ho, Anita. 2008. "Relational Autonomy or Undue Pressure? Family's Role in Medical Decision-Making." *Scandinavian Journal of Caring Sciences* 22: 128–35.

Jamieson, Lynne. 1998. *Intimacy: Personal Relationships in Modern Societies.* Cambridge, UK: Polity Press.

Kinjo, Takanobu, and Masahiro Morioka. 2011. "Narrative Responsibility and Moral Dilemma: A Case Study of a Family's Decision About a Brain-Dead Daughter." *Theoretical Medicine and Bioethics* 32: 91–99.

Lawler, Steph. 2008. "Stories and the Social World." In *Research Methods for Cultural Studies,* ed. Michael Pickering, 32–52. Edinburgh: Edinburgh University Press.

Levine, Carol. 2000. *Always on Call: When Illness Turns Families into Caregivers.* New York: United Hospital Fund of New York.

Lindemann, Hilde. 2014. *Holding and Letting Go: The Social Practice of Personal Identities.* New York: Oxford University Press.

Lindemann, Hilde, Marian Verkerk, and Margaret Walker. 2008. *Naturalized Bioethics: Toward Responsible Knowing and Practice.* Cambridge, UK: Cambridge University Press.

Lupton, Deborah. 1995. *The Imperative of Health.* London: Sage.

McCarthy, Jane Ribbons, Rosalind Edwards, and Val Gillies. 2000. "Moral Tales of the Child and the Adult: Narratives of Contemporary Family Lives Under Changing Circumstances." *Sociology* 34: 785–803.

Morgan, David. 1996. *Family Connections.* Cambridge, UK: Polity Press.

Nelson, James Lindemann, and Hilde Lindemann Nelson. 1995. *The Patient in the Family: The Ethics of Medicine and Families.* New York: Routledge.

Okin, Susan Moller. 1989. *Justice, Gender and the Family.* New York: Basic Books.

Polletta, Francesca, Pang Ching Bobby Chen, Beth Gharrity Gardner, and Alice Motes. 2011. "The Sociology of Storytelling," *Annual Review of Sociology* 37: 109–30.

Richardson, Diane. 2005. "Desiring Sameness? The Rise of a Neoliberal Politics of Normalisation." *Antipode* 37: 515–35.

Riessman, Catherine Kohler. 1993. *Narrative Analysis.* Newbury Park, CA: Sage.

Rose, Nicholas. 2006. *The Politics of Life Itself: Biomedicine, Power, and Subjectivity in the Twenty-First Century.* Princeton, NJ: Princeton University Press.

Strathern, Marilyn. 1992. *After Nature: English Kinship in the Late Twentieth Century.* Cambridge, UK: Cambridge University Press.

Taylor, Yvette. 2009. *Lesbian and Gay Parenting: Securing Social and Educational Capital.* Basingstoke, UK: Palgrave Macmillan.

Verkerk, Marian, Janice McLaughlin, Hilde Lindemann, Jackie Leach Scully, Ulrik Khilbom, Jamie Nelson, and Jacqueline Chin. 2015. "Where Families and Health Care Meet." *Journal of Medical Ethics* 41(2): 183–85.

Walby, Sylvia. 1997. *Gender Transformations.* London: Routledge.

Weeks, Jeffery, Brian Heaphy, and Catherine Donovan. 2001. *Same Sex Intimacies: Families of Choice and Other Life Experiments.* London: Routledge.

Chapter 1

Why Families Matter

HILDE LINDEMANN

This chapter explores the significance for healthcare and for treatment decisions of patients' close relationships. Beginning with the idea that these relationships have a special role in forming and maintaining the set of interconnected narratives that constitutes the identities of the people within them, I explore both how these relationships can sustain people and how they may damage them, especially when grave or chronic illness puts the relationship under pressure. I'll start with reminders of the functions of families that are sometimes forgotten in healthcare contexts. By identifying some of these functions, we can get a better sense of the responsibilities that arise from close familial or family-like relationships, and what can be at stake if families don't meet them. At the same time, I'll map the practices of responsibility that arise from these relationships, attending to the narratives that purport to justify or contest various assignments of responsibility. I close by examining how insight into practices of forming and maintaining family members' identities can help us to a better understanding of what kind of pull even the bare genetic tie between people might have.

As a preface to this discussion, three general remarks about families are in order. First, while much of the literature in bioethics on family caregiving has assumed that families are valuable for what they know about the patient and the sort of care they give, little has been said about families' crucial function in forming and maintaining the identities of their members. This chapter is largely intended to remedy that failure. Second, it is often assumed that families are nothing more than the sum of their individual members, and that they have no identity apart from that. I argue the contrary. Families are social institutions with their own histories, features, and functions. Ferdinand Schoeman calls the family an "intimate arrangement having its own goals and purposes," "an organic and enduring entity" (Schoeman 1985, 50, 54), and it is all of that. Families endure by shape-shifting: people are born into and die out of them, abandon them, enter them by marriage or other long-term commitments such as adoption, and reconfigure them by divorce and remarriage. But while families change shape over time, they also have their own distinctive characteristics. A family might, for example, be Amish or Roman Catholic, even though not everyone in the family fits that description. It might be working class or wealthy, descended from aristocracy, or Roma. Some families produce athletes in every generation, others tend toward the arts, some have a strong work ethic, and still others are blended or interracial or queer or farm or refugee.

It could still be objected that, while "family" does not refer to a sum total of the individuals who form it, it's simply shorthand for the web of *interrelationships* among those individuals, valued only insofar as the people in them are valued. But there seems to be a widely shared moral understanding that we act for the sake of the family even when we don't value some of the individuals in it. Nobody likes Grandpa Schulz very much—he is an ill-tempered bully and selfish to boot, and how Grandma Schulz puts up with him nobody can understand. But today is his birthday, and while twelve-year-old Anneliese protests that she has far more important things to do, her parents insist that she come with them to the party. "*Why* do I have to come?" Anneliese wants to know. "Because he's family."

A third prefatory point: like all human institutions, families are imperfect, and sometimes they can be dangerous, even vicious. Nor is it uncommon to find that some of our relationships inside them are unsatisfying, frustrating, odd, nasty—and these disturbing traits are often triggered precisely by other family members. This sort of experience can make the idea of family ties seem like just another discredited piety: it's to *these* people that I'm supposed to have special duties, people I never chose (except my partner), people I don't even like very much?

Coming to terms with this tension between family intuitions and family experience is in general important for living a coherent human life. Given developments in healthcare practice and policy, it takes on a certain urgency: both the growing successes and the growing expenses of contemporary medicine put families squarely on the spot to provide everything from knowledge of what the patient would have wanted, to increasingly sophisticated healthcare services, to a liver lobe or kidney. Virtually all of this progressive recruitment of family members is predicated on the idea that family connections are morally important in a variety of relevant ways, yet the question of how and why they are morally important is largely unexplored. Indeed, a primary reason for this book's existence is to arrive at a better understanding of the caring responsibilities arising from these connections. But if familial connections are not, or are no longer, the basis of special responsibilities and prerogatives, then mining families for sacrificial care would be just another form of exploitation, based on biological realities that have no moral purchase. It's the burden of this chapter to show why that isn't so.

I. FAMILIAL FUNCTIONS: IDENTITY FORMATION AND MAINTENANCE

"Persons," Annette Baier once remarked, "essentially are *second* persons who grow up with other persons" (Baier 1985, 84). This is a claim that human selves exist and act in webs of relationships with other human selves. And if it is true, as I believe it is, it means that persons are not isolated, atomic individuals. Rather, they come to be persons through their relationships with other persons. As I understand it, personhood is a social practice consisting of four necessary elements: (1) a human being has sufficient mental activity to constitute a personality; (2) aspects of this personality are sustained and expressed bodily; (3) other persons recognize it as the expression of a personality; and (4) they respond to what they see. *Recognition* and *response* are often a matter of understanding who someone is and treating them accordingly (cf. Strawson 1962). These understandings consist, first, of a web of stories we weave around our own or someone else's most important acts, experiences, characteristics, roles, relationships, and commitments. The narrative tissue formed in this way constitutes a personal identity, which plays a crucial role in the practice of personhood. And it consists, second, of a set of bodily behaviors that is similar among the family members—the way they go about things, what and how they eat and prepare for their comfort, and the way they talk and act with each other.

Our personal identities fuel the practice because they indicate who we are with respect to other persons and in that way they are *normative*: they guide not only how we are supposed to treat those others, but also how we are supposed to conduct ourselves. Our families initiate us into personhood when we are very young. Indeed, often pregnant women begin calling their fetuses into personhood before they are born (cf. Schües 2016, 111f). They do this by talking to the fetus, giving it a nickname, posting the fetal ultrasound image on Facebook, putting baby clothes in the drawer, and in other ways acting as if it were already the child that will soon be born. Fathers, grandparents, and other close relatives may call to the fetus too. And once the fetus becomes a born child, the child's intimate others *hold* her in personhood by acting on the narratives they use to recognize and respond to various aspects of the child's personality (Lindemann 2014). It's usually only when a child has no family or the family refuses its responsibilities to love and nurture the child that this holding is done solely by external caregivers. Often, the work of holding is done by family members and external caregivers alike—a baby in a neonatal intensive care unit, for example, is held by its parents and the NICU staff, and young children may be held, both physically and in personhood, by family members and daycare workers or teachers. An important function of families, then—even if it isn't generally talked about in these terms—is calling their new members into personhood and holding them there.

Families of origin, however they are formed, tend to do this identity-work better than others because familial relationships—at least, the ones we are considering here—are relationships of ongoing intimacy. This is a conceptual claim: intimate relationships, whether loving or hateful, fearful or kind, have a profound and lasting effect on the people within them because they are tightly woven, usually for many years, into the fabric of their everyday lives. Such relationships typically call on people to take up reciprocal identities. You are my sister, so I am your sister, and in that respect my identity and yours are intermingled. The people in intimate relationships are not interchangeable; they can't be replaced by similarly qualified people, which is to say that who the person is, in all her particularity, always matters. And just as intimacy implies nonfungibility, so the love and friendship that characterize positive intimacy imply partiality: the people we love are the ones we single out specially for care and concern, because that is part of what it is to love. Families, then, insofar as they are small-scale structures of enduring intimacy, are the social arrangement best suited for close-up work, and that is why they have a special importance in shaping and maintaining selves.

Holding can be done well or badly, better or worse. And while family members sometimes feel they aren't doing it correctly, there are moral criteria to measure this by. Done well, holding a family member supports her in the creation and maintenance of a personal identity that allows her to flourish individually and in her interactions with others—it helps preserve her integrity. Done badly, the person is held in invidious, destructive narratives and comportment. Some such narratives identify the social group to which the person belongs as socially and morally inferior, and in that way the stories uphold abusive power relations between "us" and "them." In other cases, people are held in narratives that restrict their ability to grow well, preventing them from moving on fully to identities that do. Sometimes—for example, in the case of a trans or gay person—the family altogether refuses the stories that depict the person as she understands herself to be, so that her attempts to express herself get limited or no uptake, with what may be catastrophic results (Lindemann 2014).

As the children in the family grow, they learn the recognition and response that allow them to participate more fully in the practice of personhood, and at the same time, their world widens to include people outside their families and other care providers. If all goes well, they will become adept at contributing to the upkeep and maintenance of their own identities, in addition to holding others in theirs.

Notice how identity formation isn't just a matter of seeing accurately who someone is and treating her accordingly. By acting on the stories they use to identify the person, families can sometimes turn her into the person they understand her to be. If, for example, the family has a very conservative view of what women are, it may see a daughter as the kind of person who is supposed to cultivate her looks and her social popularity, but not have any further ambitions. And if it acts on those narratives by which it identifies their daughter she may turn into just the shallow sort of woman the family expected her to be. Similarly, if a family's stories of who a particular man is consist largely of representations of his stupidity and worthlessness, it can damage the son's identity quite badly—perhaps even beyond repair.

Because human beings are so malleable, I submit that families have a strong moral responsibility to exercise their function of holding them. Again, I understand "family" as more than the sum of the people within it, but here I stress its *agency*. Families, taken as social units, are moral agents in the same way that corporations or nation-states are. They hold their members well by recognizing them via stories that are accurate but that also keep open their future field of action so that they can live properly. Of course, that future field can't be wide open—families must necessarily encumber their members with a language and therefore a certain way of thinking, with relationships the person never consented to, with social and moral and perhaps religious values that are part of the family's way of life. But what families must not do is stunt their members' lives by crippling their self-conception or corrupting their moral agency.

In his book *Responsibility and the Limits of Evil*, Gary Watson (1988, 269–73) asks us to consider the case of Robert Harris. When aged twenty-five, on July 5, 1978, he saw two sixteen-year-old boys eating fast food in a parking lot, forced them into their own car at gunpoint, had them drive to a canyon, and after promising he'd let them go, shot them as they were running away, firing into their bodies multiple times until he finally killed them. Then he laughed, spun his rifle in the air, drove back to a friend's house, and finished the dead boys' lunch. Convicted and sentenced to death, he was so obnoxious on Death Row that the other inmates looked forward to his execution. But his older sister Barbara told interviewers that Robert's whole life had been marked by violence, beginning with his premature birth, triggered by his father's kicking his mother in the stomach in a drunken rage. The father, an alcoholic, was convicted of sexually molesting his two daughters, while the mother, also an alcoholic, rejected Robert and blamed him for all her troubles. His mother would kick him when, as a toddler, he came to her for affection; once his father threw a bottle at him so hard it broke, cutting his face badly. After he stole a car at the age of fourteen and was sentenced to a federal juvenile detention center, he was raped several times and tried to kill himself twice. Here is a case of a family doing a miserable job of holding one of its own in personhood, and as no one else did any better, he became morally stunted. The harm to people whose families barely hold them in personhood is certainly not always this extreme (Barbara is a case in point), but everyone requires loving, intimate relationships with persons if they are to live functioning lives themselves. What might, then, be a simple family function that one could fulfill or choose to leave undischarged becomes a moral responsibility because the stakes of not discharging it properly are so high.

When an adult has a serious setback at work, is going through a divorce, has lost a loved one, or is suffering from an illness so grave that it threatens his sense of who he is, he too may need to be held as only intimate others can hold him. And once again, intimates can do this best if they love and care especially about him. A spouse, adult child, or best friend who declined to help the person maintain his sense of self when his identity is threatened would have to have a very good reason to refuse. If they didn't, they would be morally culpable.

II. FAMILIAL FUNCTIONS: CARING FOR ONE ANOTHER

A second feature of families is that they care for their own. This function too gives rise to normative expectations: it's not just that families do this, but that they must and should do this. And again, the assignment of responsibility can be justified by the harm to the person in need of care if her family abdicates this responsibility. Because family members are supposed to love and support each other, their failure to do so inflicts suffering. The people who are supposed to take you in when you need them have abandoned you, turned their backs on you. You may be able to rely on the kindness of strangers, and the strangers may be very kind indeed, but it just isn't the same thing. Relationships of partiality such as ties of family or friendship keep people from being alone in the world, and alone is not a good thing to be when one is vulnerable and in need of care.

When one member of the family is down with a bad cold or flu, a spouse or parent or partner is expected, absent a good excuse, to provide aspirin, a hot toddy, and sympathy. When grandfather needs to be taken to the doctor, the default presumption is that if a family member is available to take him, she must take time off from her other duties and do so. Often, though, the caring responsibilities—typically assigned to the women in the family—are much greater than that. Family members are usually the first people a patient turns to when in need of a donated kidney, for example. If a family member is chronically ill, the others may be required to provide high-tech treatments, such as ventilator care or dialysis, that can be given at home. And when a family member is hospitalized, the others are expected to show up at the bedside to make sure the patient is getting adequate care.

That two-thirds of this unpaid care is given by women (Feinberg et al. 2011) raises questions of gender justice that will be addressed in a later chapter, but a good portion of it *must* be given by the person who is giving it, because it can't be given in the same way or to the same effect by anybody else. The reason has, once again, to do with the identity-work that is carried out physically in relationships of intimacy. A backrub given to a hospitalized patient by a nurse just isn't the same as a backrub given by a partner, because the partner's backrub conveys her special love, care, and concern—or at least, it does so in a family that functions well enough for partners to love each other. In giving the backrub, a partner is saying something about her own identity and the identity of her partner in relation to her.

When you are hospitalized for, say, cardiac bypass surgery, you may well suffer in Eric Cassell's sense of suffering. In his widely known article "The Nature of Suffering and the Goals of Medicine," Cassell defined suffering as "the state of severe distress associated with events that threaten the intactness of the person" (Cassell 1982, 639; see also Frank 1997). It is awareness of the disintegration, or the danger of disintegration, of one's sense of self. I part company with Cassell in that I believe there are many different kinds of suffering, but if your suffering consists of a threat to your identity, then a professional caregiver can only do so much to hold you in it. Far better is an old friend, a partner, a grown child, or other person who is close to you and has been holding you well in your identity for a long time. The difficulty, of course, is that not all intimates hold well. If your suffering is caused by your family in the first place, you may require a psychiatrist, psychoanalyst, minister, or social worker to help you repair the deformity to your identity.

As the discussion in this chapter is intended to demonstrate, the ethics we develop in this book is quite distinct from healthcare ethics, feminist ethics, or an ethic of care, even though we draw on many of the resources those approaches offer. What makes an ethics of families distinctive is that it theorizes relationships characterized by ongoing intimacy and partiality among people who are not interchangeable, and is very much centered on the practices of responsibility arising from these relationships. From that ethical perspective, decently functioning families matter because people matter: intimate familial relationships give us our earliest selves and our intimates continue to hold us in our identities—if not perfectly, then often well enough—throughout our lives. So necessary is this identity-work that when a person isn't so held, her growth is stunted, her life is impoverished, and, in the worst cases, she is not able to become a responsible member of society.

III. THE FAMILY UNDER STRESS

Serious illness puts pressure not only on individual family members but also on the family itself. The care of an acutely ill person requires the family to channel many of its resources toward a single member—an arrangement that can usually be sustained for a while but that cannot continue indefinitely while the other members do without. Illness disrupts ordinary familial functions and, if it is serious enough, threatens to break the family altogether. The inability to give familial care in a hospital setting, even when the family recognizes the need for professional help and is grateful for it, may leave family members feeling helpless and at a loss, frustrated by not being able to do what they do best.

It's not only the patient who experiences upheaval in times of serious illness. When a family's primary caregiver must spend every spare moment at the hospital, the family's young children or frail elderly relatives may find themselves less well protected than they are in happier times. They may be frightened by the long absences, unsettled by the change in their routines, less well supervised by people not thoroughly familiar with their needs and proclivities, more prone to engage in dangerous activities. At the same time, the caregiver may feel guilty that she can't be at home, worried about the children's well-being, and frustrated by her inability to look after frail elders who need her. Neighbors or family friends can go some distance toward taking the caregiver's place at home, but unlike professionals who can be replaced by equally qualified others, family members are not interchangeable, as children in particular know only too well.

All that is bad enough, but even the most well-meaning health professionals and bioethicists, who care about families but don't well understand how families matter, or who counts as family, or what's important about what families do, can make a bad situation even worse. Healthcare systems tend to treat families of patients primarily as sources of unpaid care or as repositories of the patient's preferences. When a baby born at 25 weeks' gestation is discharged from the NICU that has saved her life but left her with serious damage to lungs and brain, neonatologists may take it for granted that her family will provide the years of intensive care that will now be required. Family members with no medical training may be called on to learn how to insert a nasogastric tube or perform high-frequency chest wall oscillation, or to devote significant amounts of time providing physiotherapy. And if a kidney or liver lobe is required, healthcare providers may assume that family members will just naturally volunteer.

This nonchalant attitude toward families is arguably born of nothing worse than misunderstanding—or forgetting—what families are for. Another, more pernicious attitude arises out of the clash between healthcare ethics, which is patient-centered and individualistic, and the ethics of families, which is neither. In decently functioning families, where the ethos is much more communal and relational, people will sometimes behave in ways that, from a professional, patient-centered perspective, may seem flat-out immoral. And bioethicists trained in the impartialist, individualist moral theories originally designed to govern interactions in the public sphere have been deeply suspicious of families as well (Nelson and Nelson 1995). As a result, there is what amounts to a default setting of distrust, a presumption on the part of clinicians and bioethicists that a family is just as likely as not to be neglectful, abusive, or selfish. A wife's decision not to visit her husband every day because her energy and attention are also required at home can be seen by the staff as callous, or possibly even neglectful. A daughter's insistence that her dying mother's intensive care be forgone so that the family will not lose all their savings can be greeted with suspicions of elder abuse. A family member who lives far away but is actively involved in the patient's care may be greeted by suspicion on the part of the healthcare team because she can't be on the spot. A family's request for growth attenuation therapy for a profoundly impaired child can be construed by health professionals as a sign that the family is too lazy and selfish to provide respectful care, rather than recognizing that the procedure would enhance the child's participation in family life. It is not that families should always prevail in such disputes. My point is merely that the expression of a distinct, family-oriented perspective should also be seen and supported by professional caregivers. Such a perspective is not in itself illegitimate, undermining familial claims to care. But for a family the issue is often one of balancing out the conflicting needs of its members.

This distrust can add to the strain families are already under, posing a threat to their identities. It can call into question everything that is valuable about them, casting doubt on how well they function, how adequately they love, and whether they are doing the patient good. When coupled with greatly heightened demands on families' capacity for care, this attitude on the part of clinicians, as bolstered by bioethicists, can damage families' own sense of what they are and why that matters. Like the people within them, families under pressure need to be held in their identities by caring others who recognize what is valuable about them and treat them on the basis of that recognition. Otherwise, they are at risk of losing their integrity, perhaps to the point where they cease to be families at all.

IV. THE LIMITS OF RESPONSIBILITY

To conclude this chapter, I want to take a look at the moral pull, if any, exerted by the bare existence of a close biological connection.

Most people tend to think that being closely related to others—being someone's sister or brother, mother or father, to take clear examples—gives us reasons to respond to their wants and needs in a special way: we're disposed to act for them out of love, or for their sake. But philosophy hasn't been very helpful at justifying special responsibilities to family members. For instance, accounts of love, even familial love, often stress that feelings aren't under our control and so can't be seen as something for whose presence or absence we can be held responsible. Moral agency is therefore taken to be a matter of reasons, not feelings, and the sorts of reasons philosophers have offered for our responsibilities to others don't distinguish between strangers and close kin. They largely reduce to such concepts as "easy rescue" (the beneficiary has everything to gain, the helper nothing to lose) or "compensatory justice" (I have wronged or harmed someone and now owe her something to mitigate the damage I caused, or have received benefits beyond my due and my acts ought to reflect that), and, most typically, voluntary and informed *consent* (I promised to help or willingly assumed a certain social role).

Those sorts of reasons, however, don't seem to explain in full the special responsibilities we have toward people we appropriately identify as family. Many of us share strong intuitions that we owe our children much more than "easy rescue," and our duties to our parents are greater than would be explained by any damage we caused them. Nor does it seem that consent is doing very much of the work here: defeasibly, anyway, I owe my sister regard and support even though her being my sister has nothing to do with my having consented to anything.

Where there is a lengthy shared history between people, everything that they've gone through together can obscure how much moral pull is exerted by the sole fact of the familial connection. As Samuel Scheffler observes,

The more closely a person's reasons are seen as linked to his existing desires and motivations, the less scope there will be for dis-
tinguishing between the relationships that he has reason to value
and the relationships that he actually does value. On the other
hand, the less closely reasons are thought of as tied to existing
desires, the more room there will be to draw such distinctions.
(Scheffler 1997, 200)

So Jamie Nelson and I (Lindemann and Nelson 2014) considered two people who are complete strangers to one another: half-
brothers, living on opposite sides of the country. Perhaps, when the
mother of one boy became pregnant, her boyfriend broke up with
her and moved far away, but later married and had another child.
Perhaps the boys' mothers purchased sperm from the same vendor.
Tell the story as you like, but however they came into being, each
grew up knowing nothing of the other's existence.

Now in his early forties, the one who lives in New York—we'll
call him Ned—has just received a diagnosis of acute myeloid leu-
kemia. He is about to face his first round of chemotherapy, and
his doctor asks if he has any family members who might be interested in donating bone marrow. His seventy-year-old mother vol-
unteers but isn't histocompatible; he has no first cousins. It's then
that Ned learns he has a half-brother. His mother, we will say, tells
him the name of the sperm bank she used and from there he is
able to trace Sam, one of the donor offspring, to his home in Santa
Barbara.

The knowledge that he has a sibling changes how Ned understands himself; it's a small but significant addendum to who he takes
himself to be. The tissue of stories that constitute his self-conception
have long included the narrative of how he came into existence, so he's
always assumed, as a logical possibility if nothing more, that he might
have some sisters or brothers somewhere. But the identification of

a specific person as an actual half-brother shifts something. There's a person out there in the world who maybe looks a little like him, shares the same bloodline, is a part of his family tree. That fact adds substance to the background against which he lives his life; it enriches his sense of belonging to *these* people, being part of *this* family. Here is someone he can ask for help in getting his cancer into remission. He picks up the phone.

Does the bare biological connection between Ned and Sam give Ned's request slightly more moral pull on Sam? Would Sam be doing something at least a little wrong if, by treating the request as if it had been made by a complete stranger, he failed to recognize Ned as his brother? That he and Ned are related is at the very least an *intelligible* reason for Sam to act.

Suppose Sam wakes up the morning after Ned's call and says to his partner, Beth, "I'm going to do it—I'll get tested."

Beth, who knows how much Sam hates hospitals in general and dislikes being stuck by needles in particular, stares at him in disbelief. "Why on earth would you do that?"

"He's my brother," Sam replies.

Beth could of course push back ("What do you mean, 'brother'? He's just some East Coaster who happens to share a couple of genes with you"), but it isn't as though Sam said something like, "I had that dream about the tuna again." Sam's reply is intelligible, it seems, in that it gestures toward something important about how Sam understands himself and the responsibilities he sees arising from that self-conception.

By the same token, Ned's response would be intelligible should he feel hurt if Sam dismissed his request as coming from a total stranger. Ned's reaction of course, isn't determinative; he's a highly interested party, after all, and he would now have to look elsewhere for the bone marrow he needs. But added to this disappointment would be another that involves his identity: Sam wouldn't be recognizing that he and Ned are connected in a way that's importantly implicated in who they have each turned out to be.

That these responses would be intelligible, however, doesn't yet show that they're justifiable. To show that, we've got to find something in Ned's call on Sam that gives it prescriptive force.

On some analyses—Robert Goodin's (1997), Margaret Urban Walker's (1998), Marian Verkerk's (2012)—vulnerability is a key consideration in understanding special responsibility: roughly, we have special responsibilities to those whose interests are vulnerable to our actions and choices. So we might consider the argument that Ned is especially vulnerable to Sam's response to him. Not all vulnerabilities are equally salient, though. If I were particularly hurt by your failure to lend me money because, say, we both happen to be able to wiggle our ears and that biological fact strikes me as crucial, my idiosyncratic vulnerability would not be your problem.

Is the bare biological tie between Ned and Sam just as irrelevant from a moral point of view as a shared ability to wiggle one's ears? We can imagine someone who thinks so kindly explaining Ned's mistake: he has failed to distinguish between the genetic and the social sense of *brother*. The social sense does, according to this person, give rise to justifiable normative expectations, but genes are just genes, and no prerogatives or responsibilities attach to them. Ned has merely committed the error of transferring the moral penumbra surrounding the social sense of *brother* to the genetic sense, where it doesn't belong.

That explanation seems unsatisfactory. The connection between Ned and Sam isn't "simply biological," if that phrase suggests facts unmoored from human practices and feelings. Common attitudes and actions strongly testify to the depth of importance people assign to the biological dimension of family-making: consider Ned's and Sam's own mothers' desire to have children of their bodies. Indeed, most human societies have organized the nurture, protection, and socialization of offspring around that "simply biological" connection. We might perhaps be able to imagine other arrangements—say, the one that Plato had in mind for the Guardians of the Republic, where children are reared in common with no special attachments to or claims on any particular elders, and no distinction made between genetic siblings and others of their cohort. I'm suspicious of this, though. Had Plato himself ever been pregnant, he might not so easily have dismissed the intensity and duration of the physical intimacy between the gestating woman and the fetus she was calling into personhood. That's a tie that can be broken, of course, but there seems no good reason to break it routinely as an established social practice, as doing so is bound to violate the feelings of love and protection most parents have for their offspring. As well, some other way would have to be found to give children the identities that connect them to the past as well as singling them out specially from all others of their own generation.

In any case, that's not how we do it. The general social practice in families is to assign responsibilities and make people accountable to one another on the basis of genetic ties *as well as* the ties by which people bind themselves voluntarily. And in an era permeated with the fantasy that all our obligations are a function of our choices, the small moral tug exerted by the biological tie serves as a useful reminder that we aren't connected to others only as we choose to be, but are rather inextricably and variously and essentially bound up with other selves, including those with whose bodies we share a narrative of origin.

It's not easy to see this aspect of familial responsibilities unless one has a clear sense of what families are and why they matter. They don't, of course, matter to everybody. Yet everybody has, at one time or another, relied on the love, care, and identity-work of intimate others. Individual ethics and family ethics may clash; practically this clash can be meaningful. Here I've only been able to sketch out very roughly the moral implications of intimacy: how people's reliance on intimate others for identity formation gives rise to responsibilities of holding and care, why it matters that people in intimate relationships aren't interchangeable, why these relationships are necessarily partial, and why familial identity-work is particularly important to patients in times of serious illness. Clinicians and the bioethicists who work with them will find these reminders useful as they try to navigate the increasingly complex interactions between families and healthcare. And heeding those reminders, after all, is what an ethics of families is all about.

ACKNOWLEDGMENTS

Hearty thanks to Christina Schües for her hard work on this chapter, and to Jamie Nelson for helping me think through the "bare genetic ties" problem.

REFERENCES

Baier, Annette. 1985. "Theory and Reflective Practices." In *Postures of the Mind: Essays on Mind and Morals*, 207–27. Minneapolis: University of Minnesota Press.

Cassell, Eric. 1982. "The Nature of Suffering and the Goals of Medicine." *New England Journal of Medicine* 306: 639–45.

Feinberg, Lynn, Susan C. Reinhard, Ari Houser, and Rita Choula. "Valuing the Invaluable: 2011 Update, the Growing Contributions and Costs of Family Caregiving." AARP Public Policy Institute. https://assets.aarp.org/rgcenter/ppi/ltc/i51-caregiving.pdf, accessed 16 November 2018.

Goodin, Robert. 1997. *Protecting the Vulnerable*. Chicago: University of Chicago Press.

Lindemann, Hilde. 2014. *Holding and Letting Go: The Social Practice of Personal Identities*. New York: Oxford University Press.

Lindemann, Hilde, and James Lindemann Nelson. 2014. "The Surrogate's Authority." *Journal of Philosophy and Medicine* 39: 161–68.

Nelson, James, and Hilde Lindemann Nelson. 1995. *The Patient in the Family: An Ethics of Medicine and Families*. New York: Routledge.

Scheffler, Samuel. 1997. "Relationships and Responsibilities." *Philosophical Review* 92(3): 443.

Schoeman, Ferdinand. 1985. "Parental Discretion and Children's Rights: Background and Implications for Medical Decision-Making." *Journal of Medicine and Philosophy* 10: 45–61.

Schües, Christina. 2016. "Birth." In *Routledge Companion to Philosophy of Medicine*, ed. Miriam Solomon, Jeremy R. Simon, and Harold Kincaid, 103–14. New York: Routledge.

Strawson, Peter F. 1962. "Freedom and Resentment." *Proceedings of the British Academy* 48: 1–25.

Verkerk, Marian. 2012. "Ethics of Care in Family and Health Care." Unpublished paper.

Walker, Margaret Urban. 1998. *Moral Understandings*. New York: Routledge.

Watson, Gary. 1988. *Responsibility, Character, and the Emotions: New Essays in Moral Psychology*. New York: Cambridge University Press.

Lesbian Parents' Search for the "Right Way" to Disclose Donor Conception to Their Children

VEERLE PROVOOST

This case provides a concrete illustration of the importance of drawing relationality into healthcare, for which a case is made in Chapter 1. It will do so by exemplifying how a bioethics approach that merely protects the rights and interests of individuals is inapt as it comes to capturing the full picture of how decisions—in this case related to reproduction and reproductive medical treatment—are made within families. This case describes lesbian family initiators' experiences of constructing and narrating their family story around the conception of their children. The case is supported by empirical data, in particular data from a Belgian study that investigated the meanings of genetic and non-genetic parenthood for families using gamete donation.[1] For that study, interviews had been conducted with lesbian couples who just started treatment, as well as lesbian parents and their children seven to ten years after treatment (Wyverkens et al. 2014, 1249). All lesbian couples in the study used sperm from an anonymous donor. Current legislation in Belgium is based on donor anonymity but also allows non-anonymous donation when both donor and recipients give their prior agreement. Recently, non-genetic mothers have been granted the same legal status as fathers in a heterosexual relationship. This means that an adoption procedure is no longer required.

I. DISCLOSURE IN THE MIDST OF UNCERTAINTY ABOUT BEING RECOGNIZED AS A FAMILY

Couples who reproduce via donor conception need to allow others into the private sphere of reproduction. They are, after all, using the material of a third party.[2] Moreover, when the setting of the conception is a fertility clinic—in contrast to at-home donor insemination—medical professionals will also enter more centrally into their conception story.

Since research about the well-being of parents and children in lesbian-headed families has indicated that these families do not face more problems in terms of child well-being and psychological adjustment than more traditional families (Brewaeys 2001, 44; Van Parys et al. 2016, 140), the research focus has shifted to family communication about the donor conception (Wyverkens et al. 2015, 1223). The latter category of studies have revealed at least two misconceptions in the literature. First, it has long been wrongly presumed that for lesbian parents the disclosure of donor conception to their children would somehow be evident because it is obvious that the sperm that helped create their children came from outside the couple (Van Parys et al. 2016, 140). Second, contrary to the fact that the disclosure is often studied as a one-time event, it has been shown to happen over a longer period of time and in a bidirectional way. The story is thus not merely told by parents to their children at a particular moment in time. In contrast, it is constructed in a process of gradually molding the family tale, a process in which all family members actively take part (Van Parys et al. 2016, 150; Wyverkens et al. 2014, 1252; Nordqvist 2013, 13).

Overall, the couples we interviewed were positive about the care they received from the medical staff and had a high level of confidence in them. However, before the onset of treatment, the aspiring parents were anxious about how they would be judged by the professionals—the gatekeepers to their treatment—and whether they would be considered good enough parents to be accepted for treatment (Ravelingien et al. 2015, 596). The fear of these parents-to-be was about being set aside as a particular type of family, fundamentally different from other families, and because of that perhaps not worthy of the full title of family. They particularly feared the first meeting with the counselor. Their fear was about being addressed as a kind of family in need of special scrutiny. Even though they later felt relieved about the nature of the consultation, the couples appeared to adopt a subordinate position toward the clinic and the medical staff throughout their treatment (Ravelingien et al. 2015, 602). They were thankful for the opportunity to start a family and consciously tried avoid being "difficult patients" (e.g., by avoiding tough questions). While they acknowledged their lack of control in the donor selection process, they (partly) withdrew from informed decision making and actively downplayed initial wishes or concerns related to donor selection (Ravelingien et al. 2015, 597).

II. KINSHIP (RE)CONSTRUCTION WITHIN A GENETICIZED WORLD

Part of the aspiring parents' accommodating attitude can be explained in the context of a geneticized society. In the family narratives the parents construct, they have to deal with several challenges, for which the literature on kinship (re)construction provides a framework for understanding (Nordqvist 2014, 10)—for instance, the lack of a genetic link between one of the parents and the child and the knowledge that their child is genetically linked to a person outside the family. The genetic link between the donor and their child appeared to be a significant element, specifically in the parents' fears that the donor—due to this genetic link—could be a potential intruder in their family life, an intruder who would violate their privacy and threaten the position of the non-genetic parent (Wyverkens et al. 2014, 1252). In their communication with the child, most of the lesbian parents we studied clearly differentiated between a donor and a father and presented the sperm donor as not a member of the family (Van Parys et al. 2016, 147). They presented him as an instrument necessary to achieve their goal, thereby minimizing the importance of the genetic link between the child and the donor. However, apart from differentiating from those who are not kin, these parents also brought kinship into existence—for instance, through stressing their own resemblance with the children (Wyverkens et al. 2014, 1252).

III. DOING THE RIGHT THING FOR THE CHILD REQUIRES DOING THE RIGHT THING FOR THE FAMILY

Irrespective of the diversity of family communication approaches about the donor conception, lesbian couples in our interview study were inspired by a shared motive when dealing with questions about disclosure of donor conception: they wanted to act in the child's best interests (Van Parys et al. 2016, 143). To ensure that, these parents' first concern was generating and maintaining good relationships within the family. In their view, these relationships created a safe environment for both parents and children to share information about the form and origin of their family. They thought that, rather than the mere fact of being informed, the amount of information shared, or the manner of informing, it was the flourishing of the family and the family relations that was important. Their broader view on their child's best interests (as embedded within those of the family) contrasts with a too-exclusive focus on the welfare of the child that is often presumed in the debate on how the parents should take on their parental responsibilities. A view of the child's interests as disconnected from those of the family in which it is situated and on which it depends for its flourishing is regularly seen in the debate over openness and secrecy about the donor conception status. There, it is often stated that the truth should be revealed to the child because it is in the best interests of the child. Apart from the fact that there is no evidence supporting this claim (Pennings 2017), separating the child's interests from those of her family members, in this case her parents, could lead to more harm than good. There are parents who feel threatened by the idea that the donor would start playing a prominent role in the life of their child and who fear being viewed as not a full or a true parent by their child. Imposing on these parents the idea that they should be open in their child's best interests ignores the stress and fears this might give rise to for the parent and, as a consequence, the negative effects on the child of being raised by a parent who feels she lacks the status, social recognition, and perhaps because of that (even simply the feeling of) parental competence.

IV. WHEN PROFESSIONALS ENTER THE FAMILY

When aspiring parents entered the clinic, they also entered a specific type of relationship with the medical staff. As described in the section "Disclosure in the Midst of Uncertainty About Being

Recognized as a Family," the couples, as the receivers of treatment, adopted an accommodating attitude, downplaying initial concerns (Ravelingien et al. 2015, 597). The way the couples dealt with professional advice about the disclosure of the donor conception status to their child also stood in sharp contrast to their own views on what was best for their child and their family. The parents' perception that there was a "right way" to disclose was based on their recollection of what the counselor had advised them to do (for instance, regarding strategies to answer the child's questions in light of the age of the child). The parents' response to that perceived advice was associated with feelings of insecurity and a lack of self-confidence on the one hand and a sense of enormous responsibility for doing the right thing and avoiding harm to their child on the other. These feelings of insecurity and lack of self-confidence should be viewed in the context of lesbian couples' awareness that they will create a "different" type of family, one in which there are two mothers and no father. As will be described in Chapter 2, the search for an adequate approach to relationality in healthcare should take into account the risk of "validating a particular set of relationships" as standard or "the ones that are valued." The lesbian couples in our study were highly sensible of this (perceived) lack of recognition. They sometimes even classified their own relationship as deviant and found it understandable that their wish for a child was perceived by others as less "full-fledged." Some parents clearly feared what could go wrong in their (nonstandard) families, for instance because of offering information in a way that was not suitable to the child's developmental age, and they were highly motivated to follow professional advice about the "right way" to disclose. As one woman remarked, "They [at the hospital] just told us that there is one thing you should be careful about and that is that you never answer more than what they [the children] are asking for" (Van Parys et al. 2016, 145). The couples' dependency on professional advice is situated within their search for recognition and their longing to be valued as a true family. To "earn" this recognition, they want to do whatever they can to safeguard the interests of their child and so prove that they as a couple are worthy of having children. This explains their accommodating attitude toward professionals and their advice. Although it should be noted that professional intervention should not be viewed as problematic as such, the effect of such intervention will also be influenced by the relations between patients and professionals. At least in the perception of these lesbian couples, the professionals possess knowledge about how to disclose in the right way, and hence how to safeguard their child's best interests.

In their attempts to do it "right," some parents held on so strongly to the advice they were given by the staff at the fertility clinic that they displayed a rather rigid approach toward handling their child's questions. On the whole, this meant that they did not answer the child's questions as they would do in relation to other topics: constructing stories not for the child but with the child,[3] allowing creativity and inaccuracy, using elements that are not necessarily consistent or constant over time, and, especially, based on their own view of what was good for the family. Instead of answering their child's questions and explaining even difficult things in a language that is comprehensible for the child, as we would do when explaining that milk is not made in factories, we noticed that some parents answered their child's questions like "Do I have a daddy?" very briefly with merely "No, you do not have a daddy." The idea behind this response was that everything that was not strictly an answer to the question could harm their child because it could entail information that the child was not "developmentally ready for."

Even more, when describing the counselors' perceived advice, the focus was solely on the child (for instance, the right time in a child's life) and not on the family as a whole as they described their own view.

As explained in Chapter 1, the stories people tell about their relationships not only express how these relationships contribute to the identity of a person but are also actively used to sustain that identity as something shaped by and embedded within the family. The stories of our interviewees about the disclosure of donor conception to their children are striking illustrations of this "work that relationships do" (Chapter 2). In one family, for instance, the parents made scrapbooks about the conception for each of their children (who were all donor conceived). These books were not merely "finished products" made by the parents for the children; they were actively used by the family to continuously reconfirm the importance of (the making of) the family. The story was one of hopes and fears but also of efforts (going to the clinic, undergoing treatment, supporting each other as a couple, etc.). This story of actively building a family was used not merely for storytelling and bonding in a way bedtime stories can be used or to be treasured as a memory. It did much more than that. By repeatedly telling the story and emphasizing the story's main ingredients—longing for the child, the intention toward creating the child, the effort and time invested in the creation of the child—it became a tool for actively incorporating the child's identity within the family. Moreover, by presenting these books to others outside the family (as, in this case, the interviewer), these ingredients were used to gain social recognition as a family.

V. FAMILIES AFFECTED BY THE NORMATIVITY OF MEDICAL PRACTICE

The findings of our study shed light on how lesbian couples experience constructing and narrating their family story around the donor conception of their children and how these stories were actively used to give emphasis to the family relationships and further shape and strengthen them. Apart from the importance of the relational context of the family in how disclosure stories are made and told, the relations between the patients and the professionals are important in how the disclosure will be shaped. In this, we see an example of how *experiences themselves are already responsive and selective procedures to the practices and to their underlying and sometimes hidden norms.*

Even when counselors adhere to nondirective forms of counseling, we should be aware of how the content of that counseling is perceived in the eyes of the patients. By the very invitation to see the counselor, the message is given that these patients lack some form of knowledge or skills that will be provided during counseling. However well meant, we are signaling that medical professionals, and to an extent the society at large, have doubts about their parenting qualities and therefore consider this necessary for them. This indicates that it may be so much more difficult for professionals to be nondirective (their patients believe that there is one correct way to disclose) than has been presumed. Furthermore, the professionals' counseling may not be tailored to how parents actually manage their parental responsibilities. The current debate among psychologists and medical professionals about the presumed "right of the child to know her genetic forebears" shows that these professionals still think that parents (should) hold the well-being of their children as a principal goal, detached from goals relating to the family in general. It has already been shown that such default assumptions could be what stand in the way of effectively responding to parents' and families' needs in a health-related context (Verkerk et al. 2015, 184).

At least we should bear in mind that policies are full of normative content and that professionals, when giving advice, infiltrate the family far more that we might have anticipated. We need to reflect critically on the extent to which we will allow our hospital policies to confirm geneticized views on family formation and to scrutinize lesbian-headed families more than others, indicating that they are not acknowledged as a family in the same way as other families.

When we want to support these families in dealing with disclosure of donor conception, we should be endorsing or restoring their belief in their own abilities to create and tell stories that work for them. For this empowerment to succeed, we will first need to endorse these parents as "real" parents, not as patients who create second-best families that will be in need of professional advice. This should be the starting point for any intervention aimed at empowering parents to disclose their child's donor conception status in a way they feel comfortable with, that suits their family and that allows for their children to take part in that process.

NOTES

1. This study is part of an interdisciplinary project and takes an empirical bioethics approach to parenthood after medically assisted reproduction. The study uses qualitative research methods to investigate the meanings of social and genetic parenthood as constructed and experienced by stakeholders of gamete donation (Wyverkens et al. 2014, 1249).
2. The term "third-party reproduction" is commonly used to indicate that gametes from another person than the receiving couple have been used, or that a surrogate was involved.
3. Communication about donor conception should be seen as a bidirectional rather than a one-directional process (Van Parys et al. 2016, 150).

REFERENCES

Brewaeys, Anne. 2001. "Review: Parent– Child Relationships and Child Development in Donor Insemination Families." *Human Reproduction Update* 7: 38–46.

Nordqvist, Petra. 2014. "Bringing Kinship into Being: Connectedness, Donor Conception and Lesbian Parenthood." *Sociology* 48(2): 268–83.

Pennings, Guido. 2017. "Disclosure of Donor Conception, Age of Disclosure and the Well-Being of Donor Offspring." *Human Reproduction* 32(5): 969–73.

Ravelingien, An, Veerle Provoost, Elia Wyverkens, Ann Buysse, Petra De Sutter, and Guido Pennings. 2015. "Lesbian Couples' Views About and Experiences of Not Being Able to Choose Their Sperm Donor." *Culture, Health & Sexuality* 17(5): 592–606.

Van Parys, Hanna, Elia Wyverkens, Veerle Provoost, Petra De Sutter, Guido Pennings, and Ann Buysse. 2016. "Family Communication About Donor Conception: A Qualitative Study with Lesbian Parents." *Family Process* 55: 139–54.

Verkerk, Marian A., Hilde Lindemann, Janice McLaughlin, Jackie Leach Scully, Ulrik Kihlbom, Jamie Nelson, and Jacqueline Chin. 2015. "Where Families and Healthcare Meet." *Journal of Medical Ethics* 41(2): 183–85.

Wyverkens, Elia, Veerle Provoost, An Ravelingien, Petra De Sutter, Guido Pennings, and Ann Buysse. 2014. "Beyond Sperm Cells: A Qualitative Study on Constructed Meanings of the Sperm Donor in Lesbian Families." *Human Reproduction* 29(6): 1248–54.

Wyverkens, Elia, Hanna Van Parys, and Ann Buysse. 2015. "Experiences of Family Relationships Among Donor-Conceived Families: A Meta-Ethnography." *Qualitative Health Research* 25(9): 1223–40.

Chapter 2

Recognizing Family

JANICE MCLAUGHLIN

Relational approaches, such as those associated with feminist explorations of "relational autonomy" (Beever and Morar 2016; Hendl 2016; Marway and Widdows 2015), are increasingly present within bioethics. Such approaches counter bioethical frameworks that emphasize the needs and interests of the individual within healthcare with an approach that seeks to understand people's capacities and choices as embedded in the relationships that shape them as a person (Lindemann et al. 2008). Rather than see the people around someone in need of health or social support as either a resource to be utilized or a problem to be overcome, this form of ethical evaluation sees the incorporation of the relational life of an individual as central to the provision of appropriate care. Of particular importance has been family as a key aspect of relational life (Crouch and Elliot 1999). In the context of healthcare, this prioritization is understandable given that it is often the family of people who are ill with whom healthcare practitioners come into contact and who appear to generate the kind of tensions they turn to bioethicists to help resolve. It also seems reasonable to claim that the majority of people would say that they spend much of their lives in the company of others—others they speak of as family. Nevertheless, as bioethical writers have sought to give value to the familial location of people, there has always been a tension about what families are being spoken of and what qualities are being given to them. The tension revolves around whether advocating for family to be acknowledged leads to validating particular templates of what a family both looks like and does, as the cornerstone of the case that they should have a special place in health and social care. The risk in falling into or implying such a template is the exclusion of other forms of relational life that people may or may not define as familial but that they wish to see recognized in their journey through health and social care.

This chapter seeks to explore some of the complexities involved in recognizing family and draws from a range of work interrogating what is meant by the term. It does so to support the bioethical concern with the importance of relationships to selfhood, of which family is a key form, while also attesting to the politics and risks of such a move. The overall argument is that we need to take care around the recognition dynamics involved in advocating that particular kinds of relationship are important to acknowledge in health and social care. This argument is worked through by exploring two important terms in the debates on family, *vulnerability* and *value*, and by layering a sociological account of both into their role in validating a relational/ family approach to selfhood and health and social care ethics. Before doing so, I will lay out the case made for drawing relationality into health and social care.

I. PATIENT IN THE FAMILY

The Patient in the Family (Nelson and Nelson 1995), first published in 1995, remains a key articulation of the need to recognize that individuals are sustained over a lifetime by important relationships in their lives, of which family is central. Relationships such as family matter because they inform who a person is and what that person will want at times of illness and death, and therefore they need to be brought into the engagement between patient and healthcare practitioner. The relationships that people are in throughout their lives inform not just their values and concerns but also their sense of self. People do not just think practically about how what happens to them affects others; they think of others because those others sustain them through events such as ill health. Close relationships are aspects of what makes people who they are; close relationships also help people make sense of such events. The individuals within such relationships matter to such an extent that it is crucial that the effects on those individuals are part of how people make decisions about what is best for them. As Ho (2008, 131) has also argued:

> Family members, who are constants in a changing plethora of health professionals and whose relations with the patient have been part of the individual's identity, are reminders that the patient is not a mere collection of dysfunctional body parts that require professional intervention, but a moral agent with full histories and important relationships. In this context of patienthood, dependency on family involvement may preserve rather than violate autonomous agency—it can help to maintain a range of identifications that can promote the patient's own sense of integrity and worth.

As was noted in *The Patient in the Family*, the work that relationships do to sustain people's identity occurs, at least in part, through the stories people tell about those relationships. These stories are an important route through which people can develop their sense of who they are, through the histories they are connected to and the opportunities created for them to find their place within such stories:

Families link us to a particular past and particular future, as they root us in their traditions and affirm for us what is worth living and working for. The family reconfigures as the people within it grow, but the story that is lived out within the successive configurations preserves its continuity. This ongoing tale, to which each individual's life-story contributes a narrative thread, makes an enormous contribution both to our sense of who we are, and to our sense of why it matters who we are. (Nelson and Nelson 1995, 95)

More recently Lindemann (2014) has written of the importance of such relationships and the stories told of and by them as something that "holds" us in our identities. They do so by enabling us to be who we believe ourselves to be; to have the personhood that bioethics and health and social care aim to protect and care for us. Health and social care practitioners should appreciate the importance of family, for which a more detailed case is made in Chapter 1 of this collection, because what happens when people are ill will be made sense of by them in light of their relational context, including the stories told then and in the future about who they are within the relationships that matter to them.

The arguments of bioethical approaches advocating relationality overlap with other theoretical moves in social theory to decenter the individual. For example, feminist social theory accounts of citizenship and care have called for society to recognize the value and intrinsic nature of our interdependence on the others we live with and through (Brown 1993; Lister 1997; Phillips 1993; Sevenhuijsen 1998; Tronto 1993). Such work emphasizes how our identity is interwoven in the lives of others, and that it is this embeddedness that is the source of our agency—agency that is positioned as political and collective rather than individual and self-interested (Marway and

Widdows 2015; Rudy 1999; Yuval-Davis 1997, 2011). Ho usefully summarizes such approaches as advocating that "our self is constituted to an important degree by relations with and responsibilities towards our intimates, and these relations and the welfare of our loved ones may be more significant than the interests of any individual self in isolation" (2008, 131). Connected to this work have emerged similar arguments around disability that seek to fracture the assumed boundary between those who care and those in need of care—the ill or disabled—by exploring the ways in which society is made up of "reciprocal dependencies" (Fine and Glendinning 2005, 616) and "mutual vulnerability" (Baier 1995). Again what is emphasized is that by depending on others, we all become capable of exercising our capacities (Donchin 2001; B. E. Gibson 2006; B. E. Gibson et al. 2012; Levine 2005). What perhaps distinguishes the bioethical work on relationality from feminist social theory and disability studies work exploring the concept is the focus on the relational tie. While the interdependencies within families are not ignored in these other relational accounts, the focus instead is on the broader set of relations that form across a range of spaces and connections.

It would, however, be a mistake to imply too strong a distinction between feminist social theory or disability studies work on relationality and the ideas emerging in bioethics. Bioethical ideas working with relationality do acknowledge three caveats to their focus on family as important to selfhood, caveats that are linked to the importance of feminist ideas to their development. First, it acknowledges that not all families, particularly those we are born into or find ourselves within as children (families of origin), do in their actual everyday practices manage to hold us in our identity. Through lack of care or interest, or through inaction or rejection, families can fail to provide the relational context that sustains us (Hardwig 1990). This includes their refusal to acknowledge what it is we articulate as being the core of our selfhood—the classic and still present example being the rejection of the gay child. The cost to individuals when a family acts in this way is evidence for bioethical accounts of relationality of the importance of that relationship to our identity. It matters to us when families fail to value our selfhood. Second, there is space within the notion of holding us as we are for also appreciating that our identity is not unchanging. Instead, our relationships are factors in the emergent nature of our identity, including families' "letting us go" (Lindemann 2014) so we can explore different versions of who we want to be in the company of others. Finally, the exploration of family has always been inclusive to varied forms of family formation, acknowledging as it does that universalizing or essentializing tales of family rooted in a focus on reproduction or origin do not grasp the many ways people narrate and enact ties as central to them via a language of family. Bioethical work on relationality points to the ways in which those rejected by families of origin may then go on to articulate other close relationships, which may be within a household and monogamous or may not, as family—for example, the long history of "families of choice" or "fictive kin" in gay and lesbian communities (Weeks et al. 2001).

So the issue is how to draw relationality into health and social care in a way that sees recognition of family as likely to be important to people but that also avoids some of the risks that come with validating a particular set of relationships as the ones that are valued. What I would like to suggest is that sociological approaches to narrative, identity, and family can help bioethics avoid unintentionally implying any fixed quality to the nature of family, while also still arguing for its particular importance. This work aims to think about how existing narratives about family influence how people both navigate and speak of a range of relationships that are important to them and why they do want to claim them as family.

II. NARRATIVE FRAMINGS OF FAMILY

Sociological approaches to narrative acknowledge, as do bioethics accounts of relationality, that the stories we tell and how we can tell them are crucial to the formation of individual and group identity (Lawler 2008). Where they differ perhaps is in the greater emphasis given in sociological work on the social and cultural sources of people's narratives of who they are and who they belong with. Narratives are thought of as the framing that ensures stories are tellable because they conform to the style of other stories (Maines and Bridger 2001). The existing framings people draw from so that their stories are understood are embedded in social and cultural relations (Keightley 2008). Given that there are inequalities in social relations and norms, such inequalities will filter into what narratives are available, accepted, and understood for people to tell stories of who they are. If stories are to help people form identities, others must understand and accept the stories. If this means that the available narratives limit what can be told of who someone is, then they inhibit the ability of people to tell stories through a framing that makes sense to them. Equally, if they try to make the story meaningful to themselves and their identity, their story may be misunderstood because it does not fit within existing narrative framings. For example, someone who is a parent of a child not biologically related to them, whom they co-parent with their same-sex partner, may struggle to have their story recognized by others because the existing narrative framings of who a parent is do not help them tell their story.

As this example indicates, this way of thinking about the social importance of narrative can be (and is) used to think about how and why people tell stories about relationships as familial and the social implications of the narratives available to tell those stories (Franklin and McKinnon 2001; Jamieson 1998; Smart 2011). Accounts of some families as being natural, or the foundation of society, or constituted through the bloodline are narratives that inform how people tell stories about their families, whether or not they are recognizable within such existing narratives (Carsten 2000, 2004; Gillis 1996). These existing narratives produce a need to think about how to carve a tellable story around family forms that do not equate to such recognizable narratives: some have an easier story to tell about what connects them to others. Writers working within the sociology of family argue that people who live within intimate ties that they recognize as familial, but that fall outside the usual narratives, draw from existing narratives of what family is so as to ensure that others recognize them as family (Taylor 2009). Through this approach, what they aim for is that their relational lives be valued by others (Finch 2007). Indeed, it may be that the term *family* itself is used because no other term exists that others recognize and through which people can easily say that it is this set of relational ties that matter to the formation of their identity.

Combining bioethical work on relationality and sociological work on narrative, identity, and family together helps ensure that even if we see particular ties narrated as familial as socially contingent, we can still conceptualize them as hugely important to someone's opportunities to develop selfhood and have that selfhood valued by others. Narrating relational ties as familial is a way to connect how we live together with others to modes of living others can recognize. This directs our gaze toward understanding how it is that the social influences relations formed as familial, what scope such relations have to have a say in health and social care contexts, and what value inheres or is given to those relations. That is, the concern for health and social care ethics should be about finding routes through which people's relational life can be acknowledged, alongside scrutinizing how and why particular familiar relations are acknowledged more than others. I want to develop this argument further across two fronts, first by exploring issues of vulnerability in people's relational lives and second by considering the harm that occurs when relational ties are misrecognized as lacking value because they do not conform to existing narratives of what families are, which are embedded in social inequalities.

III. VULNERABILITY

Bioethics accounts of relationality share sociology's interest in the influence of varied and changing social norms on the narratives people tell about family; they appreciate that family ties can take different forms and be spoken of in particular ways. However, alongside they also speak of some things that appear to exist (or should exist) in all families and that are the basis of arguing they should have privileged status in health and social care. For example, *The Patient in the Family* (Nelson and Nelson 1995) makes the case for the distinctiveness of the nonconsensual ties that families generate—and the value of such ties. If there are certain things that emerge within familial relations, then familial life (however formed) is distinct from other forms of intimate ties. It should then only be those ties containing those things that are thought of as family and recognized within health and social care. What is happening here is that the particular is acknowledged (family can be "done" in different ways) while at the same time some aspects of a good familial relationship are maintained as universal (family enables the relational self to emerge). Therefore, the social is recognized as being the particular bit, and a universal quality is protected from the influence of the social as instead an intrinsic value, which may not empirically occur in every family but is what family is capable of being. To challenge this—a little—I want to probe whether the particular can be separated from the special value family has. I do so by exploring vulnerability as another special value of family.

Family is said to produce certain vulnerabilities that develop out of the relationships that make them what they are (Cassidy 2013). If we need family to hold us in our identity, then we become vulnerable to the withholding of that validation. The closeness we share to others can be in a variety of intimate relations, but the vulnerability is the same across the relationships that we narrate as family (in a sense it is our vulnerability as adults, as well as children, to those we have a deep emotional loving connection to that leads us to speak of them as family). What also is said to follow is that because we are vulnerable to what family members may or may not do to us, there are responsibilities that follow for members to act or refrain from acting in such a way as to ensure those vulnerabilities do not generate harm. Perhaps one of the most shared and experienced vulnerabilities connected to the family is that of the child to the parent or caregiver, regardless of whether that child is biologically related or is brought into the family via other routes, such as adoption or assisted conception. In a paper arguing against children's having rights, the well-known philosopher Onora O'Neill (1988) proposes that children have specific vulnerabilities, which emerge from their unique dependency due to the simple fact that they require the care and attention of adult others:

> Younger children are completely and unavoidably dependent on those who have power over their lives. Theirs is not a dependence which has been artificially produced (although it can be artificially prolonged); nor can it be ended merely by social or political changes, nor are others reciprocally dependent on children. (1988, 461)

Based on this dependency there are a range of particular obligations placed on parents or other close family members, as well as a focus on parents or guardians having rights to make decisions on their children's behalf, rather than children themselves as having rights—this is what bioethicists refer to as parental liberty (Greenberg and Bailey 2001).

While there are ways in which children are vulnerable as children and ways in which society expects families—in particular parents (again whether biological or those who take on responsibility for a child)—to care for children, is this, or other vulnerabilities familial relations generate, enough to explain the uniqueness of family and its right to be given privileged status in health and social care? And if we do want to place such vulnerabilities at the heart of why family matters, how do we do so (can we do so?) without giving family inherent characteristics that lie beyond their social formation? I would like to argue that we can recognize the vulnerability of childhood and the importance that generates for relational ties, while also stressing the socially contingent nature of both those vulnerabilities and ties, all the way through. Such a focus on the social making of vulnerability and relational ties can help emphasize the need for both to be recognized in health and social care contexts.

Various sociology of childhood theorists argue that children's dependency is encouraged by a social world that restricts their opportunities to develop scope for agency (Archard 1993; James 1993). Social and cultural change, in the Global North at least, has extended the era of childhood and the importance of vulnerability and innocence as the markers of that childhood (Aries 1962). Writers also argue that if you look at the everyday social worlds of children, they are enacting agency in lots of ways, which the emphasis on dependency fails to recognize or appreciate (Corsaro 2005). Interestingly, those advocating for some version of children's rights (the key concept O'Neill sought to discredit in her argument for seeing childhood as inherently a time of dependency) go down the route of relational agency (Moosa-Mitha 2005). That is, within the everyday worlds of children are the relationships, to adults and children, that can enable them in the company of others to have an influence on their lives.

Children are only uniquely dependent against a template of autonomous individualism—the same individualism bioethical accounts advocating relationality argue is problematic in that it does not recognize the relational nature of our identity:

> I would re-define children's rights of freedom, in this associational sense, by examining if children are able to have a presence in the many relationships in which they participate. By presence, I mean the degree to which the voice, contribution and agency of the child is acknowledged in their many relationships. Presence, more than autonomy, acknowledges the self as relational and dialogical, thereby suggesting that it is not enough to have a voice, it is equally important to also be heard in order for one to have a presence in society. (Moosa-Mitha 2005, 381)

This concentration on recognizing what children are already part of and doing generates a more emancipatory and generous imaginary, which allows us to increase children's presence and to advocate for relational opportunities within which they can thrive. It is within relationships that children's agency can develop and grow. Such agency does not need to reach the high standards asked by those, such as O'Neill, who question children's capacity to be rights holders, while also recognizing the relational and contingent nature of all people's ability and wish to participate in things that matter to them.

If we think of children's identity and scope for agency as relational, then we can think of both their vulnerability to others and the role of family in making decisions on their behalf in a different, socially situated, way. It is within the varied social and intimate relations that children are part of that they will develop a sense of self and opportunities to express agency in their lives. Families can be important relational actors in that process, but so can friends. If friends, rather than family, help a child or young person with a chronic health problem manage the medications and lifestyle choices that can improve their quality of life, this seems a useful way to engage their relational life in reducing their vulnerability. Drawing in the importance of families and others in enabling *agency*, rather than primarily merely protecting against vulnerability, also provides an important counterbalance to notions of parental liberty. One area where this is debated is in relation to disability and medical intervention (Parens 2006).

If parents consent to surgeries for their disabled children because they want to conform to social norms, particularly around appearance, are they doing something that is in the best interests of the child, including the development of their relational agency? Focusing here on interventions linked to social norms is not to say that interventions that target alleviating pain or prolonging life are not without problems; however, here I want to concentrate on those primarily geared to responding to social contexts. Children undergo painful surgeries or physiotherapy, which take them away from their everyday life, in order to look less unusual, or to remain walking rather than using a wheelchair, even though walking will be more painful and more tiring than using assistive technology. Disability studies writers query the "clinical necessity" of such interventions and argue that they problematically send a message to children that their bodies are not acceptable (McLaughlin and Coleman-Fountain 2014). Here, it could be said that the relationship between the child and parent generates vulnerability because the child is dependent on the actions and decisions of the adult. However, this is not a vulnerability inherent in the dependency of the child to the adult. This is a vulnerability that is deeply social in that it emerges from societal discomfort with disability, which the parents may share or may think they are protecting their child from by agreeing to or advocating for surgical procedures (Ouellette 2010). The important debates that have arisen out of parental wishes to do what they think best for their disabled children cannot be divorced from the social contexts that inform those desires. It is these contexts that are informing the relations around the child in a way that confines their opportunities to develop some agency in their lives (Kerruish and McMillan 2015). The useful thing for bioethics to do here is to participate in debates about the balance between "fixing" disabled children under pressure from societal norms and querying those norms and the vulnerability they generate for disabled children and those who care for them.

IV. VALUE

Earlier in the chapter I suggested that we can draw from both relational bioethics and sociology of family to make a case that family is an important relationship to be recognized in health and social care for two reasons. First, our identity and agency is relational, and relational ties therefore should be present in health and social care situations where our identity and agency is important. Second, family is a form of relationship that is given particular value in society. It is a framing that influences people's relational ties, both how they read them and how others read them. Here I want to explore how particular types of relationship come to be given social value and what that might mean in different health and social care contexts. What I now want to suggest is that one of the key social vulnerabilities to family relations' being able to sustain their members' agency and identity is the misrecognition of those relations as being problematic in some way, as not being valuable. Linking back to narrative, I want to suggest it is those whose narratives fit less well with the standard narratives that inform societal understandings of what families are who are the most likely to be misrecognized. It is also these situated actors who are the most vulnerable to having their capacity to support relational identity and agency undermined. The implication here is that health and social care ethics should consider not just how to draw family relationships into health and social care dynamics. They should also pay attention to how to do so without replicating broader social inequalities, which lead to some familial relationships being given greater value than others (a theme picked up in the case study by Cutaş and Gheauş in Chapter 3).

Following through my interest in the importance of the social within the recognition of relationships as being familial, I want to focus on the way the social also influences how judgments get made about appropriate familial relationships. That is, a set of relationships may be recognized as familial but also judged as not "good" forms of family life. Particular forms of family relationships are judged better than others because they conform to existing narratives about what families are: based in a household, long-term, monogamous, and formed with the aim of producing and raising children. For example, in the social, political, and legal moves to recognize lesbian and gay families, various queer writers have highlighted the dominance of that heterosexual template within the law and in social approval (Richardson 2005, 2015). An important influence on practices of judgment and misrecognition is the way that economic inequalities rooted in class influence how judgments get made about different kinds of families. The types of relationships most easily recognized as both familial and valuable are those that also are associated with middle-class lives.

Various sociologists of family have pointed out that while people live and "do" family in different ways, those familial forms that are seen as the norm are also those associated with particular social values, which are themselves associated with particular groups in society (Morgan 1996; Smart and Neal 1998). These associations are used to judge alternative forms of family, which are then deemed as acceptable only if they enact the norms of "normal families." Penalties follow for those who fail to enact the "right" values in their familial practices. The significance of cultural recognition and governance dynamics around families is seen most clearly when scrutiny falls on those deemed to have values that fall outside acceptability (Lawler 2002). Not all family narratives, histories, and relations are given equal value in all areas of society. Certain families seeking to establish their familial affinities struggle to respond to preexisting narratives, which assert they are of little or no value, because of their association with a range of troubling social categories associated problematically with poverty: the young single-mother family, the family "living on benefits/social security," the family with children from multiple previous (or ongoing) relationships. Finch's (2007) work on family narratives emphasizes the use people, particularly those living in poverty, make of displays of family life and ritual in order that others recognize their relationships as familial and appropriate. The work such families do comes from an awareness that the negative consequences are high for failure to conform.

Class is drawn into such accounts because it is argued that the varied forms of familial relationships most regularly judged as disreputable are linked to working-class lives, while the norms associated with the "good" family life are assumed to be more present in middle-class lives. It is the middle class who are said to know how to "do" family, in particular to raise children with the correct values and aspirations for adult life. For example, in the UK governments from the 1990s onwards have spoken of "troubled families" as those in working-class locations who fail to pass on the correct values about work and aspiration to their children, and who are defined as the source of social problems in their location. Such families are explicitly marked as troubled by the ways in which they differ from other families through the varied forms of familial life they enact: for example, teenage pregnancy and multiple pregnancies with absent fathers (MacDonald et al. 2014). One problem with the notion of the "troubled family" is the pretty sketchy evidence that such families exist and that they are the source of the complex systemic problems faced in such areas (Levitas 2012); another problem—my focus here—is the cultural, class-based judgments being made through the associations between varied family forms, social location, and lack of value.

Skeggs (1997), drawing from Bourdieu (1989, 1996), argues that social inequalities are the source of the different values given to different modes of life in society, but also that those inequalities are then validated and sustained through those values. Various cultural and social institutions produce "regimes of value" (Skeggs 2011) that are associated with particular class groups that then validate the boundaries of acceptability associated with different groups. This enables particular groups to be judged as both lacking in value and causing their own social marginalization. Through such dynamics certain groups are recognized as "subjects of value" while others are not. In contemporary cultural values, driven by the dominance of the individualism of neoliberalism, one of the main subjects that lack value in the contemporary imaginary are those whose class position, varied practices, and embodiments mark them as "non-propelling, non-future accruing subject[s]" (Skeggs and Loveday 2012, 475)—that is, those who are apparently not doing enough to become the self-reliant individual good citizen. Such values are said to be embedded in working-class communities and to be reproduced via family relations that pass such values down multiple generations (McLaughlin 2015). In this way family ties and the stories such communities tell of their family history and location are placed by others in a narrative framing that misrecognizes those ties as inherently problematic. Skeggs and Loveday argue that those tarred by narratives that trouble their position in society produce their own counter-narratives, often by valuing the very relationships said to define their lack of respectability, but what they cannot guarantee is that such counter-values will be recognized by others. Therefore, Skeggs and Loveday ask,

"How do we comprehend what value means to those symbolically positioned to have no value, the wrong culture and defective psychology, who are held morally responsible for all the structural inequalities they inherit and by which they are positioned?" (2012, 486–7). While the focus here on class may (the emphasis is on *may*) locate this discussion within the importance class has to continued inequalities in the UK, what travels is that in different locations there are social narratives that judge some families as less valued than others. These narratives link the poverty such families experience to the way they live their family lives, and such judgments become a vehicle to blame them for their social position. In the context of the US, the most obvious comparison is the vilified figure of the African American single mother receiving welfare benefits (Fraser and Gordon 1997).

The question is this: What does this matter to wanting to see families recognized within health and social care? The risk I see is that this move of recognition could become another opportunity for the social inequalities, which lie behind the legitimation of certain families, to influence which families are provided with the opportunity to have a say in what happens in health and social care. This happens easily when judgments are made about which families have the capacity to be involved because they appear to have the values others associate with families living the "right" kind of life in the "right" kind of way, with the resources that enable them to interact appropriately with health and social care practitioners. As I mentioned earlier in the chapter in relation to understanding the sources of vulnerability in childhood, what this requires from bioethics is that when calling for families to be present in health and social care, equal attention must be given to the social, cultural, political, and economic dynamics influencing the narrative framings available through which families are recognized as valuable enough to engage with.

V. CONCLUSION

In a call for a "postmodern bioethics," Gibson argues that the focus of bioethics should be "adopting a critical perspective towards healthcare, acknowledging that practices invariably privilege some people over others" (2015, 175). As someone from outside the tradition of bioethics, it is not for me to say what kind of bioethics could help resolve the challenges of contemporary health and social care for the people who work and are treated there. However, it does seem useful when exploring those challenges to think of the sometimes inadvertent and at other times systemic ways in which certain groups are privileged. The dynamic of privileging I have been interested in here revolves around recognition. When it is proposed that relationships matter to individuals and that they should therefore matter within health and social care, an important step is taken. The next step is critically reflecting on which relationships are then said to matter and how. Families are complex social institutions whose shape, values, and influence on people's lives and identities are mediated by the social, cultural, political, and economic conditions within which they form. Many people live their lives within varied forms of intimate life, which they demarcate as familial. That they do so says something about the importance of family, but it also says something about the dominance of the narrative of family as something that shapes how people speak of and enact their relational life. Therefore, in drawing relationality into health and social care and proposing that family is a particularly significant form of relationality, it is important to remain conscious of the social in influencing the framing of the relational as familial—and the significance of that framing for leading both to vulnerability and to misrecognition of which relations are valuable enough to acknowledge.

REFERENCES

Archard, David. 1993. *Children: Rights and Childhood*. London: Routledge.

Aries, Philippe. 1962. *Centuries of Childhood*. London: Jonathan Cape.

Baier, Annette. 1997. "Trust and Antitrust." In *Feminist Social Thought: A Reader*, ed. Diana Tietjens Meyers, 604–29. London: Routledge.

Beever, Jonathan, and Nicolae Morar. 2016. "The Porosity of Autonomy: Social and Biological Constitution of the Patient in Biomedicine." *American Journal of Bioethics* 16(2): 34–45.

Bourdieu, Pierre. 1989. *Distinction: A Social Critique of the Judgement of Taste*. London: Routledge.

Bourdieu, Pierre. 1996. "On the Family as a Realized Category." *Theory, Culture & Society* 13(3): 19–26.

Brown, Wendy. 1993. "Wounded Attachments." *Political Theory* 21(3): 390–410.

Carsten, Janet, ed. 2000. *Cultures of Relatedness*. Cambridge, UK: Cambridge University Press.

Carsten, Janet. 2003. *After Kinship*. Cambridge, UK: Cambridge University Press.

Cassidy, Lisa. 2013. "Thoughts on the Bioethics of Estranged Biological Kin." *Hypatia: A Journal of Feminist Philosophy* 28(1): 32–48.

Corsaro, William. 2005. *The Sociology of Childhood*. Thousand Oaks, CA: Pine Forge Press.

Crouch, Robert, and Carl Elliot. 1999. "Moral Agency and the Family: The Case of Living Related Organ Transplantation." *Cambridge Quarterly of Healthcare Ethics* 8: 275–87.

Donchin, Anne. 2001. "Understanding Autonomy Relationally: Toward a Reconfiguration of Bioethical Principles." *Journal of Medical Philosophy* 26: 365–386.

Finch, Janet. 2007. "Displaying Families." *Sociology* 41(1): 65–81.

Fine, Michael, and Caroline Glendinning. 2005. "Dependence, Independence or Inter-Dependence? Revisiting the Concepts of 'Care' and 'Dependency.'" *Ageing & Society* 25: 601–21.

Franklin, Sarah, and Susan McKinnon. 2001. "Relative Values: Reconfiguring Kinship Studies." In *Relative Values: Reconfiguring Kinship Studies*, ed. Sarah Franklin and Susan McKinnon, 1–28. Durham, NC: Duke University Press.

Fraser, Nancy, and Linda Gordon. 1997. "'A Genealogy of 'Dependency': Tracing a Keyword of the U.S. Welfare State." In *Justice Interruptus*, ed. Nancy Fraser, 121–50. London: Routledge.

Gibson, Barbara E. 2006. "Disability, Connectivity and Transgressing the Autonomous Body." *Journal of Medical Humanities* 27: 187–96.

Gibson, Barbara E., Franco A. Carnevale, and Gillian King. 2012. "'This Is My Way': Reimagining Disability, In/Dependence and Interconnectedness of Persons and Assistive Technologies." *Disability and Rehabilitation* 34(22): 1894–99.

Gibson, David. 2015. "Toward a Postmodern Bioethics." *Cambridge Quarterly of Healthcare Ethics* 24(2): 175–84.

Gillis, John R. 1996. *A World of Their Own Making*. Boston, MA: Harvard University Press.

Greenberg, Aaron S., and J. Michael Bailey. 2001. "Parental Selection of Children's Sexual Orientation." *Archives of Sexual Behavior* 30(4): 423–37.

Hardwig, John. 1990. "What About the Family?" *Hastings Center Report* 20: 5–10.

Hendl, Tereza. 2016. "The Complexity of Relational Autonomy: A Holistic Approach to Embodiment." *American Journal of Bioethics* 16(2): 63–65.

Ho, Anita. 2008. "Relational Autonomy or Undue Pressure? Family's Role in Medical Decision-Making." *Scandinavian Journal of Caring Sciences* 22(1): 128–35.

James, Alison. 1993. *Childhood Identities: Self and Social Relationships*. Edinburgh: Edinburgh University Press.

Jamieson, Lyne. 1998. *Intimacy: Personal Relationships in Modern Societies*. Cambridge, UK: Polity Press.

Keightley, Emily. 2008. "Engaging with Memory." In *Research Methods for Cultural Studies*, ed. Michael Pickering, 175–92. Edinburgh: Edinburgh University Press.

Kerruish, Nicola, and John McMillan. 2015. "Parental Reasoning About Growth Attenuation Therapy: Report of a Single-Case Study." *Journal of Medical Ethics* 41(9): 745–49.

Lawler, Stephanie. 2002. "Mobs and Monsters: Independent Man Meets Paulsgrove Woman." *Feminist Theory* 3(1): 103–13.

Lawler, Stephanie. 2008. "Stories and the Social World." In *Research Methods for Cultural Studies*, ed. Michael Pickering, 32–52. Edinburgh: Edinburgh University Press.

Levine, Carol. 2005. "Acceptance, Avoidance, and Ambiguity: Conflicting Social Values About Childhood Disability." *Kennedy Institute of Ethics Journal* 15(4): 371–83.

Levitas, Ruth. 2012. "There May Be Trouble Ahead: What We Know About Those 120,000 'Troubled' Families." *Poverty and Social Exclusion in the UK*, Policy Response No 3: http://www.poverty.ac.uk/system/files/WP%20Policy%20 Response%20No.23-%20%20'Trouble'%20ahead%20(Levitas%20Final%20 21April2012).pdf.

Lindemann, Hilde. 2014. *Holding and Letting Go*. Oxford: Oxford University Press.

Lindenmann, Hilde, Marian Verkerk, and Margaret Walker, eds. 2008. *Naturalized Bioethics: Toward Responsible Knowing and Practice*. Cambridge, UK: Cambridge University Press.

Lister, Ruth. 1997. *Citizenship: Feminist Perspectives*. Basingstoke, UK: Macmillan.

MacDonald, Robert, Tracey Shildrick, and Andy Furlong. 2014. "In Search of 'Intergenerational Cultures of Worklessness': Hunting the Yeti and Shooting Zombies." *Critical Social Policy* 34(2): 199–220.

Maines, David, and Jeffrey Bridger. 2001. "Narrative Structures and Social Institutions." In *The Faultline of Consciousness: A View of Interactionism in Sociology*, ed. David Maines. Hawthorne, NY: Aldine de Gruyter.

Marway, Herjeet., and Helen Widdows. 2015. "Philosophical Feminist Bioethics Past, Present, and Future." *Cambridge Quarterly of Healthcare Ethics* 24(2): 165–74.

McLaughlin, Janice. 2015. "Family Ties in Genes and Stories: The Importance of Value and Recognition in the Narratives People Tell of Family." *The Sociological Review* 63(3): 626–43.

McLaughlin, Janice, and Edmund Coleman-Fountain. 2014. "The Unfinished Body: The Medical and Social Reshaping of Disabled Young Bodies." *Social Science and Medicine* 120 (November): 76–84.

Moosa-Mitha, Mehmoona. 2005. "A Difference-Centred Alternative to Theorization of Children's Citizenship Rights." *Citizenship Studies* 9(4): 369–88.

Morgan, David. 1996. *Family Connections*. Cambridge, UK: Polity Press.

Nelson, James Lindemann, and Hilde Lindemann Nelson. 1995. *The Patient in the Family: An Ethics of Medicine and Families*. New York: Routledge.

O'Neill, Onora. 1988. "Children's Rights and Children's Lives." *Ethics, Place and Environment* 98(3): 445–63.

Ouellette, Alica. 2010. "Shaping Parental Authority over Children's Bodies." *Indiana Law Journal* 85(3): 955–1002.

Parens, Erik, ed. 2006 .*Surgically Shaping Children: Technology, Ethics and the Pursuit of Normality*. Baltimore, MD: The John Hopkins University Press.

Phillips, Anne. 1993. *Democracy and Difference*. Cambridge, UK: Polity Press.

Richardson, Diane. 2005. "Desiring Sameness? The Rise of a Neoliberal Politics of Normalisation." *Antipode* 37(3): 515–35.

Richardson, Diane. 2017. "Rethinking Sexual Citizenship." *Sociology* 51(2): 208–24.

Rudy, Kathy. 1999. "Liberal Theory and Feminist Politics." *Women and Politics* 20(2): 33–57.

Sevenhuijsen, Selma. 1998. *Citizenship and the Ethics of Care*. London: Routledge.

Skeggs, Bev. 1997. *Formations of Class and Gender*. London: Sage.

Skeggs, Bev. 2011. "Imagining Personhood Differently: Person Value and Autonomist Working-Class Value Practices." *Sociological Review* 59(3): 496–513.

Skeggs, Bev, and Val Loveday. 2012. "Struggles for Value: Value Practices, Injustice, Judgment, Affect and the Idea of Class." *British Journal of Sociology* 63(3): 472–90.

Smart, Carol. 2011. "Families, Secrets and Memories." *Sociology* 45(4): 539–53.

Smart, Carol, and Bren Neal. 1998. *Family Fragments*. Cambridge, UK: Polity Press.

Taylor, Yvette. 2009. *Lesbian and Gay Parenting: Securing Social and Educational Capital*. Basingstoke, UK: Palgrave Macmillan.

Tronto, Joan.C. 1993. *Moral Boundaries: A Political Argument for an Ethic of Care.* London: Routledge.

Weeks, Jeffrey, Brian Heaphy, and Catherine Donovan. 2001. *Same Sex Intimacies: Families of Choice and Other Life Experiments.* London: Routledge.

Yuval-Davis, Nira. 1997. "Women, Citizenship and Difference." *Feminist Review* 57: 4–27.

Yuval-David, Nira. 2011. "Belonging and the Politics of Belonging." In *Contesting Recognition: Culture, Identity and Citizenship,* ed. Janice McLaughlin, Peter Phillimore, and Diane Richardson, 20–35. Basingstoke, UK: Palgrave.

The Family Imperative in Genetic Testing

LORRAINE COWLEY

The context of this case study, based on empirical qualitative research, is genetic testing for cancer susceptibility. Within genetics, information may have shared significance for family members, but not everyone necessarily has the same desire to know their genetic probability of developing cancer. Professional ethics codes in the UK dictate that genetic testing is offered as an individual choice, not a shared one (Association of Genetic Nurses and Counsellors 2016), although in practice family members may be invited to, or request, shared appointments. There are pressures around genetic testing, based on perceptions of responsibility to family, that are important to how people approach their own and others' choices in genetic testing (Cowley 2016). Family dynamics of choice can be evident to genetic counselors when family members share appointments. Here the ideal of individual choice comes into contact with pressures of family dynamics, and these may influence how people engage with choice as individuals. As a contribution to the themes of the chapter, this case study illustrates how genetic relatedness does not necessarily correlate with shared close or social relationships. It emphasizes the importance of determining which relationships matter to whom in an environment where normative assumptions about moral responsibilities to family members not only arise but are contested and justified.

I. BACKGROUND TO THE STUDY

The social research, presented for a Ph.D. degree,[1] was conducted in the UK and focused on a family known to a regional genetics service. The term *family* at this stage refers to a genetically defined kinship group as defined by the genetic family tree or "pedigree" that was constructed over decades of research into their history of early onset cancer. Prior to this social study, the family contributed to medical research that characterized one of the genes causing Lynch syndrome (LS)[2] (hMLh1) (Kolodner et al. 1995), making testing for LS possible and for the family to be the first to know their genetic risk for LS. They are distinctive when compared to others who undergo testing in contemporary genetic counseling practice.[3] Their engagement with genetic investigation began in the 1960s when their general practitioner noticed that multiple young family members developed bowel cancer. With some of the family he began a genealogical project that was continued by genetics services in the 1980s. The project linked others with cancer to the family (Dunstone and Knaggs 1972).[4] Some who were previously unaware of their biological links became known to each other through these efforts. Against this background family members had been offered genetic testing, but not all had accepted.

My research, conducted between 2007 and 2012, aimed to explore how their family's experiences with genetic investigation shaped or shifted notions of kin. In a series of narrative interviews, participants were invited to discuss their experiences of genetic testing and their

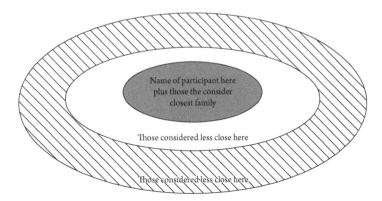

Figure 2.1 Social maps

understandings of family. The interviews were semi-structured, but interviewees' own associative trails were followed; *they* chose what to tell *me*. I used photo and graphic elicitation techniques to stimulate responses—for example, by asking them to talk about family photographs, showing them their genetic pedigree, and asking them to construct social maps (Fig. 2.1). Social maps depicted concentric circles within which participants showed who they considered to be closest family (i.e., those placed in the central circle). These narrative methods produced selective accounts, and in their selection of what to tell and with what emphasis, participants created moral identities (Cowley 2012; Singer 2004).

II. DIFFERENCES IN FAMILY REPRESENTATIONS

I compared the data from participants' social maps to their narratives about their pedigree. Within anthropology and sociology, contemporary work on kinship has highlighted two changes to our understandings of kin. The first is that patterns of kinship that are not based on biology and are instead "chosen" (e.g., families of choice, blended families, fictive kin) are increasingly visible (Finkler 2000; Weeks 2001). The second is that so-called natural biologically based families display dynamics of responsibility that also indicate the significance of negotiation and choice in their lives. However, by investigating inherited medical conditions, biomedical definitions of family, over which we have no choice, are emphasized in clinical genetics. Within medical anthropology, this emphasis is referred to as the "medicalization" of kinship (Sachs 2004), and this case study, whose focus is on understanding which relationships matter to whom, has relevance for appreciating the dynamics of family responsibility within clinical genetic practice.

The visual methodologies I deployed elicited rich narratives about participants' social practices and meanings of "family." Each participant's representation of family was shown to be different. For example, among three sibling pairs, none reciprocated closeness on their social family maps (Fig. 2.2); the number of people included in each person's innermost circle ranged between two and thirty; many social maps, with the exception of parents and children, did not have any correspondence with the pedigree.

While social maps depicted who mattered most to participants, the pedigree was discussed in a different way. Participants viewed it as a means of visualizing order from apparently random or disordered social experiences. They approached the pedigree as a means of systematically discovering both social relationships and the genetic susceptibility to cancer. For example, one participant found out from the pedigree that he went to school with people who were later identified as his relatives. He talked about those people as relatives after the fact of knowing them as school acquaintances: "I wasn't aware that somewhere down the family tree they were related."

It was evident in participants' accounts, when the pedigree was shown in interviews and when they constructed their social maps,

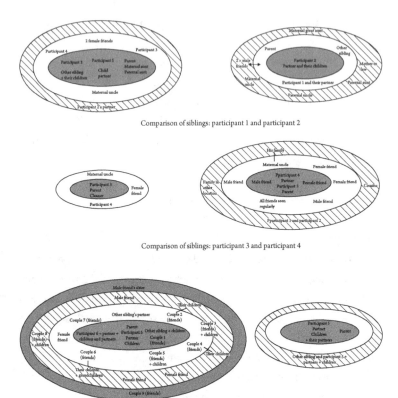

Comparison of siblings: participant 1 and participant 2

Comparison of siblings: participant 3 and participant 4

Comparison of siblings: participant 5 and participant 6

Figure 2.2 Comparison of social maps

that the medical account and each participant's perception of "family" were at one level conflicting or, at the very least, incongruent. The following quote from Gill, spoken when looking at the pedigree, illustrates this point:

> GILL: And all these people I recognize from this village (laughs).
> I don't even know them, but I recognize the names.
> ME: So do you feel that these people are your kin?
> GILL: No, no, they're just strangers.

Gill's quote was broadly typical of the reactions to the pedigree, and I did not get a sense of collective family identity in interviewees' accounts except when they discussed the medical discovery of LS.

III. ANNE'S STORY

However, for one interviewee, Anne, the genetic construction of her family tree had troubling social consequences. Anne did not include any of her biological relations on her social map, with the exception of her children and grandchildren. Unaware of the social distance between them, genetic practitioners invited Anne and her siblings, whom she had not seen for twenty years and with whom she had an acrimonious relationship, to shared appointments for genetic testing. Of her siblings, with whom she shared the appointments, Anne said, "I just don't think of them now as family, you know? Which is awful, but I don't." Of the genetic department's arrangement of a shared appointment, she said, "Well, they didn't know we all didn't speak." Genetics healthcare professionals had assumed a social relationship between siblings, and the process of genetic testing had provided three opportunities for them to share the same clinical space. Conceivably, this must have been a difficult situation for Anne and her siblings. Although not explicit in her quote, the appointments did not produce a long-lasting sense of connectedness; it lasted only the duration of the intervention and was discussed as an uncomfortable social experience, fraught with tension.

Despite medical circumstances providing the focus for bringing Anne and her siblings together, medicalization cannot seemingly impose a social connection that is not there. Within the data it was evident that kinship bonds or ties were left unchanged when participants engaged with the medical pedigree. This was most evident from the social maps. No one placed people whom they had only met as family through a medical intervention in their inner social circle or indeed anywhere on their social map. The medical construction of family in these data presented at best a potential opportunity to be curious about biological relations in a social sense, but as Lock et al. (2007) and others (Novas and Rose 2000; Rose 2007) have suggested, this was not enough to change kinship bonds or ties.

IV. MAKING MORAL CHOICES

A lack of correspondence between medical and social versions of kin has the potential to complicate any notion of shared responsibility and decision making in genetics. My research highlighted potential social harms of genetic testing for LS, both for those who decide to have a genetic test and for those who decline. The importance of lived relationships influenced the way in which responsibility to have genetic testing was understood. While having a right to choose was considered paramount by participants, those who exercised that right by choosing to decline testing were deemed to be making the "wrong" choice by those who chose to be tested. The data showed that to have a genetic test is to act on moral imperatives that framed self-identities of being a good parent, a good family member, and a good citizen. A key conclusion was that perceptions of responsibility to "family" are important to how people approach their own and others' choices in genetic testing. Choices about testing may be founded on their senses of caring for kin, fulfilling a sense of family obligations, and caring for themselves, such that declining a test would for them, and perhaps others, be seen as morally wanting. Although the decision to be tested was considered a responsibility to family and therefore an imperative, some of those who declined testing were still accepted by family members, and their act of declining a test was discursively excused or ameliorated.

Participants continually negotiated complex boundaries in making sense of their choices about closeness, who is family, who is kin, and how they understand and frame the boundaries to those for whom they, or others, believe they have responsibility. While choice was framed as an immutable right, participants discursively negotiated the boundaries of responsibility to those they call kin. These dynamics became most obvious and acute in discussions regarding family members who chose to decline testing. The ethical work that participants undertook not only to defend their own decision making but also to excuse the decisions of test decliners so that they might remain "family" was apparent. Although individuals in families may have made what were considered wrong decisions about treatment, the bonds of family relationships were negotiated and presented in ways that made unacceptable decisions possible to accept (Cowley 2016). Relevant to the context of this chapter, although participants made decisions based on shared moral understandings of family responsibility, what was not shared was agreement about who was family. There was no shared sense of a collective family identity, and given the moral landscape of decision making, this makes finding out who matters to whom central to the ethical deployment of genetic information.

V. CONCLUSION

The context of decision making about genetic susceptibility to cancer has highlighted a moral responsibility to have a genetic test. Although not explicitly narrated as a shared decision, those who decided to have a test had shared moral understandings about their decisions. I gave examples of how healthcare professionals confused medicalized versions of kin, constructed via genetic investigations, with the social realities of family. In conclusion, understanding family practices and narratives is central to decision making for individuals in genetics, where shared decision making is not brokered and sometimes the biological relationships that are medically informative are not the relationships that matter to people in a social sense. Individuals making decisions about genetic testing may or may not negotiate or share the decision-making process with all of those who will be affected by the information. The socially conceived responsibilities to "family" may or may not map to those identified by healthcare professionals as "at risk" via the genetic pedigree. Tensions are produced between what is shared between whom, and what or who matters to whom, because families' distinctive individual social practices do not correlate to the biological facts. It is these tensions that make it particularly sensitive that healthcare professionals in genetics understand the family practices of those they identify on a genetic pedigree as being at potential increased risk of cancer.

NOTES

1. Funded by Cancer Research UK—Nurses' Research Training Fellowship.
2. Those with LS have an increased lifetime risk of developing cancers of the bowel, cancers of the digestive and urinary tracts, and, in women, cancers of the endometrium and ovaries. People at increased risk are referred for bowel surveillance colonoscopies every eighteen months to two years from the age of twenty-five years. There is no proven effective surveillance for gynecological cancers. Women who have a mutation are additionally invited to discuss cancer preventive surgery (removing their ovaries and uterus) from the age of thirty-five to manage their increased risk of gynecological cancers, providing they do not want (more) children.
3. In current practice those having genetic testing might see a genetics professional up to three times over three to six months. This varies depending on local policies and practices.
4. This family has been discussed in the medical literature. Some family members have contributed to television documentaries. Care has been taken to ensure anonymity and de-identification of individuals by using pseudonyms and

de-gendering relationships within quotes. Genetics colleagues who have proof-read quotes were unable to identify participants they would usually know.

REFERENCES

Association of Genetic Nurses and Counsellors. 2016. Code of Ethics for Genetic Counsellors. http://www.agnc.org.uk, accessed May 31, 2016.

Cowley, Lorraine. 2012. *Genetics and Kinship: Finding Morality at Their Intersection.* Ph.D. thesis, Newcastle University.

Cowley, Lorraine. 2016. "What Can We Learn from Patients' Ethical Thinking About the Right 'Not to Know' in Genomics? Lessons from Cancer Genetic Testing for Genetic Counselling." *Bioethics* 30: 628–35.

Dunstone, George H., and Terence William Knaggs. 1972. "Familial Cancer of the Colon and Rectum." *Journal of Medical Genetics* 9: 451–56.

Finkler, Kaja. 2000. *Experiencing the New Genetics: Family and Kinship on the Medical Frontier.* Philadelphia: University of Pennsylvania Press.

Kolodner, Richard, Nigel Hall, James Lipford, Michael Kane, Paul Morrison, Paul Finan, John Burn, et al. 1995. "Structure of the Human MLH1 Locus and Analysis of a Large Hereditary Nonpolyposis Colorectal Carcinoma Kindred for MLH1 Mutations." *Cancer Research* 55(2): 242–48.

Lock, Margaret, Julia Freeman, Gillian Chilibeck, Briony Beveridge, and Miriam Padolsky. 2007. "Susceptibility Genes and the Question of Embodied Identity." *Medical Anthropology Quarterly* 21(3): 25676.

Novas, Carlos, and Nikolas Rose. 2000. "Genetic Risk and the Birth of the Somatic Individual." *Economy and Society* 29(4): 485–513.

Rose, Nikolas. 2007. *The Politics of Life Itself: Biomedicine, Power and Subjectivity in the Twenty-First Century.* Princeton, NJ: Princeton University Press.

Sachs, Lisbeth. 2004. "The New Age of the Molecular Family: An Anthropological View on the Medicalization of Kinship." *Scandinavian Journal of Public Health* 32(1): 24–29.

Singer, Jefferson. 2004. "Narrative Identity and Meaning Making Across the Adult Lifespan: An Introduction." *Journal of Personality* 72(3): 437–59.

Weeks, Jeffrey. 2001. "Families of Choice: The Changing Context of Non-Heterosexual Relationships in Same Sex Intimacies." In *Same Sex Intimacies: Families of Choice and Other Life Experiments*, ed. Jeffery Weeks, Brian Heaphy, and Catherine Donovan, 9–27. London: Routledge.

What Counts as a Family—
And Who Is to Decide?

MARGARETA HYDÉN

This case study seeks to explore some of the complexities involved in a child's and later a young woman's efforts to be recognized by the adult world as a human being in deep trouble. It originates from an interview with Mary, a twenty-three-year-old woman who participated in my study of social network responses to young people with health problems.[1] Since her family was the locus of her troubles, she had tried to get recognition from adults at a daycare center, from the healthcare system, from social services, at school, and finally from the Stockholm City Mission (SCM),[2] a nongovernmental organization providing help for socially vulnerable people in the city of Stockholm.

In the beginning of the interview, I gave Mary a piece of paper with an outline for a "social network map" consisting of a circle divided into four spheres representing "family," "relatives," "friends and neighbors," and "working life." I asked her to plot the people in her network and tell me how they had responded to her troubles. As it turned out, her map was sparsely inhabited. In the "family" sphere were her mother and her sister written in tiny letters and the STOCKHOLM CITY MISSION in big letters. The "friends and neighbors sphere" also had STOCKHOLM CITY MISSION written all over it, and the remaining two spheres were empty.

Mary's social network map and the narratives that accompany it challenge taken-for-granted assumptions about families, such as demographic and governmental definitions of traditional families, with members linked by blood, law, or adoption and a shared day-to-day life. Her narrative brings to the fore some essential questions for a relational bioethical approach to healthcare, such as: What counts as a family—and who is to decide? What kind of ethical dilemmas will personnel in a family-oriented healthcare system have to face if they meet children who introduce them to family forms that are not self-evident?

Mary's narrative is divided into two parts, both concerning the connection between Mary, her problems, and the responding adult world.

I. THE BROKEN CONNECTION BETWEEN CHILD AND PROBLEM

Constructing the "Problematic Child"

When I asked Mary to tell me about her social network's responses to her health problems, she started by telling me about herself as a *problematic child*. The narrative was driven forward by a series of complicating actions[3] and orientations that contained various kinds of violence:

> I was very problematic as a child. (Abstract)
> I hurt myself from an early age. At the age of four I started to bite myself, tear my hair, was very angry at everything and everyone, foremost with myself. (Complicating Action)

They noticed that at the daycare. (Orientation)

I behaved in a special way, I could scream for hours, I could bite myself, bang my head against the wall, that sort of thing. (Complicating Action)

My father was very violent. He hit me when I was little. He left when I was seven. (Orientation)

My mum was an alcoholic. She gave the impression of being very fragile. At the daycare center they felt sorry for her: "Your child is so problematic, we can understand if you are tired." (Orientation)

Then my mum began to talk about that maybe there was something wrong with me, with my head. I was sent for testing and they checked if there was something wrong with my brain, if I had some kind of diagnosis. They didn't find anything. (Complicating Action)

Then the daycare center hired an extra person to look after me. (Resolution/Coda)

A series of narratives are amalgamated into this narrative and contribute to the construction of the problematic child. There is the embodied story of a child in tremendous pain; there is the story of a fragile and probably abused mother; there is the story of the daycare center and the steps taken for dealing with a vulnerable parent and a child causing problems by her violent and deviant behavior. Finally, there is the story of the healthcare personnel engaged in examining Mary's pain in an attempt to give it meaning in the medical world (Mishler 1984). In Mary's case, the healthcare assessment suggested that her pain and suffering *could not* be understood as signs of underlying medical conditions. By assigning this meaning, the healthcare system, inextricably bound up with the medicalization of pain and suffering, played an important role in constructing the problematic child: if she was not suffering from a medical condition, she was solely problematic.

There is a big difference between *having problems* and *being problematic*. To *have problems* indicates a relation between you and your problems, and you will belong to a category everybody will inhabit from time to time. To *be problematic*, however, is not a category marked by relationships. The connection between you and your problems is broken and the problems are attributed to you as a quality or characteristic. People will view you as a person belonging to a special category of people no one wants to be in. A problematic child is predestined to engage in problematic activities and problematic relations; "non-problematic children" will be advised to avoid any closer contact.

Responsive and Responsible Responses

Responses to personal problems could be *responsive* to the emotions and needs of the person in trouble and they might be regarded as *responsible*, implying a moral imperative to reduce risk and prevent a recurrence. When the healthcare workers refrained from medicalizing Mary's problems, it could be viewed as a responsible response, given the results of the assessment, at the same time as it was not responsive to her pain and need for help. Correspondingly, when the daycare center personnel joined the mother and identified Mary as "the problematic," no room was allowed for responses to Mary's need for care. However, the discourse of the problematic gave room for some action at the daycare center that could be viewed as responsible: a child with violent and self-destructive behavior justified the employment of an extra person to deal with her, something that might reduce the risk for serious injury.

Reinforcing the "Problematic Child"

The continuation of Mary's narrative did not contain any reports of improved health. As she got older, she spent less time with her family and more time hanging out in the neighborhood. She exposed herself to the risk of being exploited sexually and becoming involved in criminal activities. She found other children who were also considered "problematic," and with them she was no longer an "other." She could escape her position as the problem, at the same time as it was reinforced by her problem lifestyle. At the age of twelve, she reached out to social services for help:

> I was twelve, almost thirteen, when I stopped going to school. I was with other kids in the same situation. I was very self-destructive, used drugs, harmed myself by cutting. I was sexually exploited by a man at the local youth club. (Orientation)
>
> I tried to change all this. (Abstract)
>
> After a fight with my mother and stepfather, I went to the social services and asked for a new place to stay because of my mum's drinking problems. (Complicating Action)
>
> They said that before they could do anything, they had to set up a meeting with my mum and me and I said NO. Then they asked me if I didn't want any help? I just ran away from them. (Complicating Action)
>
> They called my mother right away. She and my stepfather got very angry and he tried to lock me up in the wardrobe. (Complicating Action)
>
> There was a meeting at the social welfare center. (Complicating Action)
>
> My mother told the social workers that I was a problem and had been so for a long time. (Resolution/Coda)

As in the first part of the narrative, issues of responsibility and moral obligations are crosscutting elements. Since Mary was underage, the morality included her parents, in this case the mother as the custodial parent, the social services agency, and the healthcare system. The morality comprised some basic assumptions about what it means to be responsive and responsible vis-à-vis an underage family member in trouble. A key issue was the division of responsibility between the custodial parent and the social services agency.

Mary reached out to the social services agency, told them about her problems with her parents, and asked for a new place to stay. Contacting the custodial parent was the regular procedure for the social services agency concerning "problematic" young people. Their defining feature of a parent was based on *parental obligations.* Although the times we live in are marked by individualization, the Swedish social services for young people demonstrate an explicit family-of-origin profile. Confronted by a runaway youth, their pronounced objective is to "bring home" the youth and reintegrate him or her with their often sorely wounded families (Sjöblom 2004, 132). By reinforcing the mother's legal and moral obligations to control the problematic Mary, the social services agency shaped the understanding of what a family is and how it should be structured.

II. RESTORING THE BROKEN CONNECTION BETWEEN CHILD AND PROBLEM

It was a single remark from a female teacher that eventually punctured the feature of the "problematic child":

> I think it all collapsed one day. (Abstract)
> My teacher asked me why I had been late often. It seemed to have become a habit of mine. (Complicating action)
> I just broke down. I was surprised at my reaction; I was usually meeting the world with a tough "fuck off" attitude. I think

it was because she was such a nice and caring person and because she had told me so many times that I was a great and talented pupil. I couldn't stand the thought of having disappointed her. (Evaluation)

To my great surprise *she* almost broke down too! She apologized for her remark, telling me that she hadn't mean to criticize me, just wanted to help, wanted to know how I felt and what was going on. (Complicating action)

I just cried and cried. (Complicating action)

I just couldn't cope with so much kindness. (Resolution/Coda)

This episode triggered a series of responses. The teacher referred Mary to the school psychologist, who step by step built a relationship with her and addressed her as a great and talented pupil in trouble. The psychologist introduced Mary to various activities for adolescents at the SCM. People from the SCM accompanied her to the social services agency, and this time they met her with a more responsive—and responsible—attitude and she got a new place to stay. She continued to come to the SCM almost daily.

At twenty-three, Mary holds a B.A. in social sciences and plans a career in psychology. She has reconnected with her mother and sister, but she still considers the SCM her family. She visits them often, and when something important happens in her life, such as a new job or a new boyfriend, they are the first to know.

III. THE EXPANDED FAMILY AS A FAMILY FORM FOR RESTORING BROKEN CONNECTIONS

Mary's narrative contains a series of responses that reflect the adult world's understanding of responsible responsiveness, responses that were not responsive to her needs. Her network map and narratives draw our attention away from the generally adopted definitions of family as linked by blood and law and toward the *quality of relational ties* as the focal point for determining what family is—namely, *family is where there are responsive and responsible responses to the child's problems and vulnerability*. These relational ties could be established between the child and people far outside the inner circle in the network and form an expanded family, based on relations and moral obligations that are voluntarily undertaken.

IV. CAN HEALTHCARE PERSONNEL MEET THE EXPANDED FAMILY?

When it came to moral decisions about how to help her, Mary's traditional family did not serve her well. Her pain and suffering went unrecognized by her family and the surrounding adult world. It was suppressed and was never articulated until she was taken care of in a context she called "family" and I will call "an expanded family form." At the age of twelve, Mary reached out for an expansion of her family, and when some years later she got the chance, she was active in establishing an expanded family.

Can a child be entrusted with the task of identifying his or her family? I think many will answer "yes." Could that family be valid in meetings with healthcare personnel? I think many will answer "no," "maybe," or "depending on age." Some might say, "It sounds reasonable and we can work in that direction, but we cannot adopt it directly." Reasonable or not, it was the expanded family that managed to carry Mary's story, developing it and making it available for other adults with special obligations, like social services and healthcare personnel.

NOTES

1. "The Significance of Social Network's Responses to Young People's Health Problems" is a pilot study based on narrative and social network analysis of interviews with five young women, aiming to contribute to the development of a model for intervention and prevention. The Swedish Research Council for Health, Working Life, and Well-Being funded the study.
2. The Stockholm City Mission is a nongovernmental, not-for-profit organization that since 1853 has provided help to socially vulnerable people and to children, young adults, and the elderly.
3. To grasp how Mary understood how her social network had responded to her health problems, I delineated and classified the structure of the narrative. I based my analysis on the narrative structure theory developed by Labov and Waletzky (1967) and the six elements of storytelling they identified: (1) Abstract (what is the narrative about?), (2) Orientation (who or what are involved in the narrative, and when and where did it take place?), (3) Complicating Action (then what happened?), (4) Resolution (what finally happened?), (5) Evaluation (so what?), and (6) Coda (how does it all end?).

REFERENCES

Labov, W., and J. Waletzky. 1967. "Narrative Analysis." In *Essays on the Verbal and Visual Arts*, ed. J. Helm, 12–44. Seattle: University of Washington Press.

Mishler, E. G. 1984. *The Discourse of Medicine: Dialectics of Medical Interviews*. Norwood, NJ: Ablex Publishing Corporation.

Chapter 3

Negotiating Responsibilities

MARIAN A. VERKERK

One Sunday afternoon Sara got a call from her brother Vincent: "It's Mum again. She's not doing so well—her leg is getting worse and her memory is starting to go bad. The home care team says she really needs more help than they can give, so they want us to put her in the nursing home where they can take better care of her." Even though Sara and her mother live in the same town, they don't see each other very often; the last time was more than half a year ago. Still, Vincent's call was no real surprise, since the elderly woman's health had been gradually going downhill for years. But the board of the nursing home had instituted a new rule that the family must spend at least four hours a month with their relative—and Sara lived near their mother.

"It's a kind of contract, actually. We're asked to show some responsibility for Mum and in return they provide an optimal living and care environment," Vincent explained.

"So that means . . .?" asked Sara.

"Well, I live pretty far away from her. I have a demanding job and Myrna can't just walk away from the kids. You live around the corner from her and you're alone, so four hours a month doesn't seem like a lot to ask."

"But you know I hardly ever see her," Sara said. "I can't stand her—she's a totally nasty, evil person."

"I know," said Vincent, "but she's our mother, for God's sake. We're only talking about four hours a month!"

I. THE PROBLEM

The European welfare state, in which care for the elderly has become institutionalized as well as professionalized, is in financially heavy weather. The increasingly aging population, together with the decreasing number of state-supported elder care givers, makes it almost impossible to guarantee the quality of care the elderly need. Especially difficult to meet are personal attention, walks, and talks. Because professional care workers can barely meet the physical needs, other sociopsychological and existential needs cannot be addressed adequately, so relatives are sometimes asked to take care of them. In the Netherlands some nursing homes are trying to arrange a form of contract with relatives; for admission of their relative in the nursing home, the closest relatives are asked to visit their mother or father in return. But even without these kinds of contracts, there is more and more a sentiment in Western societies that the government or state does not bear the sole responsibility for care of the elderly; family care should be provided too.

The argument used is that family members have a moral responsibility to give such care. The discussion is focused on the idea that solidarity among citizens should not be guaranteed solely by governmental care but should also be promoted in other ways. The critique is that we have become too used to seeing each other as independent citizens who care for the dependent by way of governmentally guaranteed care, when we ought instead to be morally concerned about each other. We should focus more on informal and communal solidarity.

A cynical way of looking at this discussion would be that families, and probably especially women, are being exploited to keep up with the pressing needs of an aging population. And there may be some truth to this. On the other hand, there is a case to be made for family responsibility. In ethical theory, family obligations are classified as a form of special responsibility. But even if we accept the idea that there are special responsibilities in families, it's difficult to spell them out precisely. At least, it's too simple to say that because they're family, we have an obligation to care for our relatives, no matter what.

In this chapter I contend that there is a moral case to be made for family care. At least two arguments can be put forward in defense of this position: (1) there is a moral familial responsibility and (2) in taking care of a family member, a certain social good is produced that cannot be obtained otherwise. I will consider family as a caring practice in which special responsibilities are distributed and negotiated. I will also argue that although family relationships count, the history of that relationship and the particulars of the situation also count in determining the moral weight of responsibilities that we have toward each other. If and how we have a particular responsibility toward a family member, say your elderly mother or father, depends on the "moral shape" of the situation (Dancy 1993; Lindemann 2014a). Political and social considerations are also part of this "moral shape," such as considerations of justice and equity. Assigning responsibilities is only intelligible against the background of existing practices and the normative expectations arising from them, whereby these practices themselves need to be evaluated. At the end, family care will be presented as a "contested practice" in which responsibilities to care are negotiated. I will therefore conclude that a case can be made for family care, but that each case has to be considered on its own terms. I will start my argument by unpacking the concept of responsibility.

II. THE CONCEPT OF RESPONSIBILITY

When we think of responsibilities, we often think of taking care of something, or of having specific commitments toward someone that it would be morally wrong to neglect (Walker 1998). Being responsible for someone implies that we have a relationship with that person. In *Protecting the Vulnerable*, Robert Goodin has specified that relationship as a relationship of vulnerability. He therefore defines his principle of (individual) responsibilities as follows: "If A's interests are vulnerable to B's actions and choices, B has a special responsibility to protect A's interests" (Goodin 1996, 99). At the same time, this principle of vulnerability makes it clear why we aren't always responsible at all times for everyone. We are only responsible for those who are vulnerable to our actions. Goodin goes on to say that "the strength of this responsibility depends strictly upon the degree to which B can affect A's interests" (Goodin 1996, 118).

Goodin's concept of responsibility is consequentialist in character. The strength and scope of one's responsibility is dependent on the aggregate outcome for a specified class of persons. Margaret Urban Walker, however, rephrases Goodin's principle of vulnerability by introducing the condition of the *"dependency in fact"* as a necessary condition to being responsible. And so she defines "being responsible" as:

> X is vulnerable to Y in respect of N when X is actually dependent on or circumstantially dependent upon Y to secure or protect N *because* of the nature of their existing relationship, some prior agreement between them or by them, a particular causal history between them, or the fact of Y's unique proximity and capability in light of X's extreme plight. (Walker 1998, 84)

So when you took care of my children during my illness and you now need to be picked up from the dentist, I have a responsibility to do so. Or when I am the only one nearby who can help you, I am morally obliged to do so. Or, because of our existing relationship, for instance because you are my daughter, I am responsible for you. We are, each in our own way, responsible for each other, because we are vulnerable—dependent in fact—through this particular connection. And so, in line with Walker's view, I think that we can speak of "family responsibilities" as part of the special relationship we have with each other and the shared history we have. But saying that is only the beginning of the moral argument of family responsibilities.

III. BECAUSE IT'S FAMILY

I have just said that family responsibilities are special responsibilities. In other words, we have certain *pro tanto* responsibilities toward family members that we don't have toward other people. The source of these specific duties lies in the fact that we are family, which is to say that *the relationship itself* gives rise to certain responsibilities. The same thing can be said about friendship: you have certain responsibilities toward your friend, because she is your friend. When a friend needs my help and I don't respond, I'm not only neglecting my responsibilities toward her, but renouncing the friendship itself.

The simple fact that we are family gives rise to certain responsibilities toward those of our own. But in saying this, we haven't settled the matter. A first question is who counts as family and who doesn't. The mere fact of having biological kinship is not determinative. Who is to be considered a family member depends on social and cultural norms. Families are of a variety of shapes and designs (Smart and Neal 1998). While some people may have more traditional views about their obligations toward their biological family, it's likely that others will be based on contemporary notions of changing family structures, which engender different obligations to different family members.

Here, I start with the assumption that, ideally, family is the place where we take care of each other and in which we experience enduring intimacy and closeness that is different from other relationships. That place is not necessarily the nuclear family of a father, mother, and one or more children. Instead, it's the web of specific, long-term relationships in which certain unique social goods are produced and shared.

IV. WHY FAMILIES MATTER

A family is not only a practice of responsibility in which we hold each other accountable for certain things. Ideally, families are also the sites where certain social goods are distributed. In families we protect, raise, and nurture our children. The family is also the place where we have a sense of belonging. Like home, family is the place—as Robert Frost says in the *Death of the Hired Man*—"where, when you have to go there, they have to take you in." Family is also the place where I get recognized as the "daughter of." My moral identity is nurtured and acknowledged within the intimacy of the family. For example, in a family Sara is recognized as her mother's daughter, for whom the mother should care; the mother is to be blamed if she neglects or abuses her daughter. In accepting this responsibility, the mother expresses herself as Sara's mother. But at the same time, she expresses the value of the relation that she has with this child: the child is her *cherished*, or *worthless*, or *resented* daughter. This is why it is so devastating for a person when a parent disowns her. Because the self is essentially always a relational self, when her father says, "You aren't my daughter anymore," an important piece of the daughter's identity is thrown into serious confusion.

The fact that the family distributes certain social goods doesn't mean that families have primarily instrumental value. We don't value them solely for the goods they deliver. Instead, we seem to value them just because they are our families. We see them as ends in themselves (Brighouse and Swift 2007, 44–80; Lindemann, 2014b, S97–S103).

V. THE MORAL SHAPE OF FAMILY CARE

I have said that if and how you have a particular responsibility toward a family member, say your elderly mother or father, depends on the moral shape of the situation (Dancy 1993; Lindemann 2014a). Several considerations can add up to form the specific moral shape, so we may conclude that there is no actual moral responsibility to care for a family member in certain particular situations. This means that we can't speak beforehand of an all-in moral responsibility to take care of family members. In the following I reflect on several considerations that seem relevant for assessing any particular moral shape.

First, the strength of one's responsibilities as well as the content of these responsibilities seems to depend on the *nature* of the relationships that give rise to them. In the case of family, we have socially specific expectations about the responsibilities that we have toward each other as family members. These expectations vary according to time and place. What is expected from relatives in Southeast Asia is quite different from expectations in some North European countries. The expectations are often based on deeply held beliefs about the cultural and moral meaning of family life and the responsibilities connected with these.

Second, for assessing the moral weight of family responsibility, it's also important to evaluate the relationship itself. For Samuel Scheffler, whether one has special responsibilities toward other family members depends on whether one has reason to *value* this specific familial relationship. But when does one have reason to value it? Families are sometimes sites of oppression and exploitation. Abusive power relations sometimes prevail in families. Instead of being places where loved ones hold someone in her identity, families can constrict people's agency. A daughter who has always been abused by her mother doesn't have reason to value this mother–daughter relationship—but the abusive mother might very well have reason to value her relation with her daughter. And even in a case of this kind, the daughter might irrationally value this relation: one of the terrible results of parental abuse is that the child doesn't see that she is being victimized by the abuser.

In any case, relationships on Scheffler's view aren't solely up to choice. Relations are to be valued as such and not only because one chose them. As Scheffler says, although the significance of choice and consent in moral contexts is undeniable, nevertheless the moral import of our relationships to other people doesn't derive solely from our own decisions. But that doesn't necessarily imply that we have to consign ourselves to a form of social bondage. We shouldn't stay in a relationship that is characterized by exploitation and oppression. We're under no obligation to keep up relations that are degrading or demeaning, or that serve to undermine rather than to enhance human flourishing (Scheffler 1997, 205).

Third, in assessing the moral weight of caring responsibilities, it's also important to consider whether the care to be given will be appropriate and competent. If the caregivers are rushed or coping in inadequate facilities, or if they are badly trained, their charges will suffer. Leaving an incontinent elderly person in her own feces, or taking her into a public space insufficiently clothed, shames the person and takes away her dignity. It seems clear that care that undermines the self-respect of the care receiver can't ever be considered morally good care.

Fourth, family as a moral practice not only gives rise to special responsibilities but can also lead to newly experienced vulnerabilities. Some elderly parents experience more vulnerability when they become dependent on their children for care. They might appreciate the walks and the talks, but not the washing and the feeding, preferring that those be given by paid professionals. Yet in creating a new scheme of responsibilities, new vulnerabilities might also be created. Before, you weren't responsible for taking care of your mother. Now you are. It's precisely the kind of care *you* can give that makes her vulnerable in the sense that she can't get it in the same way from anyone else. And if you fail to give this care, you are accountable for your inaction, as she becomes even more vulnerable because of you. Even in an abusive familial relationship, one can feel an obligation to respond to the needs of one's mother. But there are different ways to meet those needs. It also depends on how vulnerable you would become if you cared for her.

Fifth, the political context is also relevant in assessing one's moral responsibilities toward one's family. Family care should be understood not only as a moral practice but also as a political practice. Families yield, in Walker's words, a moral geography in which we can read how and upon whom responsibilities fall. And these shared understandings are always socially and culturally determined, but also gendered and classed. Caring, as Joan Tronto points out, doesn't always function in a socially egalitarian way (Tronto 1993, 116). Considerations of justice and equality should be included in the composition of the moral shape.

VI. BACK TO THE CASE

Does this analysis drive the conclusion that Sara should spend four hours a month with her frail elderly mother? Well, maybe. There is a moral case for family care, but what it amounts to depends on several considerations. As I argued earlier in the chapter, it depends on the quality of the particular relationship between the elderly parent and his or her child. It also depends on whether this particular person is uniquely situated to take care of the elderly parent. It depends on whether the self-respect of caregiver and care receiver will be diminished if family care is given. And even when a case can be made for such care in a particular situation, issues of distributive justice still need to be addressed.

Note how Vincent and Sara negotiate who is responsible for their mother's care. Vincent urges proximity and comparative ease as reasons for Sara to take this on, while Sara points to what seems to be a history of ill feeling and possibly abusive or neglectful treatment on the part of their mother as reasons why she shouldn't have to do it. Sara may also suspect that Vincent sees her as the natural caregiver because she is a woman; as with any other healthcare practice, family care is a situated and contested practice in which power, in the guise of gender, is at play.

But Vincent isn't only appealing to Sara's gender as he negotiates this responsibility with her. He also appeals to the fact that their mother is family, drawing on widely shared normative beliefs about the responsibilities arising from that relationship. Normative expectations around family care vary from time and place and depend on deep-rooted beliefs about the cultural and moral significance of family. But not everyone reads the family's moral map the same way. That is why, often, responsibilities for care in families must be negotiated until some agreement is reached about what's there to be seen.

Care in families, then, can sometimes be a contested practice, both morally and politically, in which responsibilities must be negotiated among family members as well as between professionals and informal caretakers. It requires moral sensitivity to assess what a particular situation requires when it comes to family care.

REFERENCES

Brighouse, Harry, and Adam Swift. 2007. "Legitimate Parental Partiality." *Philosophy & Public Affairs* 37(1): 43–80.

Dancy, Jonathan. 1993. *Moral Reasons.* New York: Wiley-Blackwell.

Goodin, Robert. 1996. *Protecting the Vulnerable.* Chicago: University of Chicago Press.

Lindemann, Hilde. 2014a. *Holding and Letting Go. The Social Practice of Personal Identities.* Oxford: Oxford University Press.

Lindemann, Hilde. 2014b. "Why Families Matter." *Pediatrics* 134: S97–103.

Scheffler, Samuel. 1997. "Relationships and Responsibilities." *Philosophical Review* 92(3): 443.

Smart, Carol, and Bren Neal. 1998. *Family Fragments.* Cambridge, UK: Polity Press.

Tronto, Joan. 1993. *Moral Boundaries: A Political Argument for an Ethic of Care.* New York: Routledge.

Walker, Margaret Urban. 1998. *Moral Understandings.* New York: Routledge.

Paternal Responsibility for Children and Pediatric Hospital Policies in Romania

DANIELA CUTAŞ AND ANCA GHEAUŞ

In this brief text we look at one instance of how gender norms continue to inform institutional treatment of parents regarding care for children—specifically, how the exercise of fathers' responsibilities for their children can be discouraged or altogether blocked. Expectations about fatherhood have changed significantly in Europe in the last decades (Collier and Sheldon 2008) in the direction of closer involvement in the lives and hands-on care of their children. At the same time, moral and political philosophers have for many years been stressing the value of family relationships (see, e.g., Lindemann Nelson and Lindemann Nelson 1995), and some offer accounts of why individuals of any sex are entitled to have opportunities to develop flourishing relationships with their children (see, e.g., Brighouse and Swift 2014). State regulations increasingly support parent–child relationships independently of the relationship in which parents stand to each other (Parkinson 2011, 2006). In this way, the recognition of close father–child relationships and the encouragement of uptake and continued exercise of fathers' responsibility for their children are gaining support. This is happening to unequal degrees in various European countries. In Sweden, for example, co-parenting after the parents' separation or divorce is common and expected.[1]

According to recent changes in the Romanian civil code (Monitorul Oficial 2009) that came into force in 2011, parental authority (but not the child's residence[2]) is by default shared between post-separation parents. This is a radical change from the previous legal status quo in Romania, where divorce usually led to the loss of parental authority for one parent, generally the father. (A father's loss of authority did not also imply the end of his financial responsibilities for the children.) It is unclear to what extent the changes concerning shared parental authority are implemented, and some claim that the practice has not changed and that, in fact, children are placed with one parent who controls the access of the other parent to the child.

Post-divorce parental authority provisions represent only one important change in Romania (at least on paper). Other legislative changes encourage parents to share at least some of the parental leave: one month of leave is lost if they choose not to share it. Legislative changes such as these indicate a new direction in thinking about post-separation co-parenting, one that may conflict with individual and social practices. They also indicate a new way of thinking about the division of parental responsibilities for the provision of hands-on care to the child. The widespread practice was to delegate almost all hands-on care to mothers; new legislation nudges parents toward a more gender-balanced involvement in the life of the child.

Steps are thus clearly being taken toward a more gender-egalitarian recognition of parental rights and responsibilities. Yet, in practice, mothers and fathers do not have equal opportunities to exercise their parental responsibilities in Romania. One recent example of this in the private sector has been the decision of a major gym chain in Romania to forbid parents to use the locker rooms with children of a sex different from that of the parent and other users. This effectively prevents fathers from accompanying daughters to the gym, and mothers from accompanying sons, unless another adult of the same sex as the child can accompany them and use the locker room with the child. Instead, these parents have been invited to use the toilet as a changing room. A same-sex couple who have a young daughter has filed a complaint against the gym at the Romanian National Council against Discrimination (CNCD). Following a decision from the CNCD in favor of the parents,[3] a separate locker room for families was created in the one location where the incident took place, while all other locations still lacked any solution other than the toilet (ActiveWatch 2014).

It is not only private companies that enforce a gendered division of parental responsibilities. This case study focuses on an example of public institutions preventing fathers from exercising their parental responsibilities: pediatric hospitals.

I. THE CASE

Romanian public hospitals allow, and sometimes require, a parent to stay in hospital with their child in pediatric wards. This is done for the benefit of the child and is in line with national regulations according to which children under fourteen who are hospitalized are entitled to have one family member present for the duration of the hospitalization (Ordin. 1284/2012, Art. 5). However, not all hospitals comply consistently with these regulations. In response to a petition from parents accusing hospitals of separating them from their children, representatives of the Health Ministry and Work Ministry emphasized that the hospitalization of children younger than fourteen with a parent is "a right and not a privilege" (Agerpres.ro 2016).

At the same time, even when hospitals have been willing to comply with these regulations, they have not always done so in a gender-neutral way: only the mother can spend nights in hospital with her child. This gendered interpretation of the legal regulations has been enforced even when the father was a single parent: in the absence of a mother, another female relative may take her place. Fathers can be accommodated with their children, but only subject to availability of individual hospital rooms, which are scarce and may require parents to pay an additional fee. As a result of complaints, the CNCD ruled in 2008 (Hotărîrea nr. 649/04.12.2008) that the practice is discriminatory and that hospital managers should remove these restrictions and admit fathers who wish to accompany their children, on the same terms on which they admit mothers. These recommendations have been repeated by the CNCD in subsequent complaints against hospitals.

In response, one hospital has sued the CNCD, claiming that:

Pediatric hospitals do not have separate facilities for fathers and mothers, and in particular toilets and showers;
Pediatric hospitals have beds allocated for maternal caregivers;
There are cases in which the mothers breastfeed, and for them it is embarrassing that a man is in the room;
There is medical care in which the mother is actively involved and which is more easily accepted by the children under the supervision of the mother;
This is not the only hospital in the country that imposed this rule. (Curtea de Apel Bucuresti 2009, 1–2, our translation)

On the basis of these points, the representatives of the hospital claimed that it had not discriminated against fathers and that the decision of the CNCD should be annulled. The court rejected the complaint. The first two claims were rejected on the grounds that the law requires that parents of any sex be accommodated by hospitals when they accompany minors younger than three. Any sex-based discrimination would need to be justified by very serious reasons, which, in this case, were absent. The court also found appeal to the child's comfort requiring mothers' but not fathers' presence problematic, noting that fathers and mothers are equally entitled to parental care leave by law—and thus are entitled to develop and exercise their parental care. The fact that other hospitals had similar restrictions could not be accepted as "a justification of discrimination."

II. ANALYSIS

This case offers a rich palette of issues relevant for discussions about parental and in particular paternal rights and responsibilities in relation to children. It illustrates how the exercise of fathers' responsibilities can be discouraged or altogether prevented by public institutions. Hospitals that deny fathers' access on equal terms with mothers' access are operating on a double bias: one gender-based, favoring mothers over fathers, and the other class-based, favoring fathers who can pay additional fees for overnight accommodation over those who cannot. The practice perpetuates a gendered division of labor, whereby mothers, but not fathers, are responsible for the hands-on care for their children. Feminist scholars have been arguing for a long time that the gendered division of labor is incompatible with achieving equality of opportunity for women and men in the family and in the workplace. Therefore, policies regulating childrearing, as well as their implementation, need to make gender-egalitarian sharing of hands-on care the default option (Gheauş and Robeyns 2011).

An obvious complication arises, however, when, as a matter of practice, mothers and fathers share hands-on care for children very unequally (in spite of legislation enabling or encouraging them to be more gender-egalitarian): the longer one parent is the exclusive, or main, caregiver of a child, the more specialized she or he—usually she!—becomes. While parents of any sex can in principle be equally competent caregivers, the parent who spends considerably more time caring for a child will be increasingly better at understanding and addressing that child's needs. In this way, discouraging or outright preventing fathers from acting as hands-on carers of their children, in the name of gendered parental competence, becomes a self-fulfilling prophecy.

As we have illustrated, the transition from gender-traditional to gender-egalitarian childrearing is likely to involve costs, both for the child and for the less experienced parent. In our view, the existence of these costs does not justify the perpetuation of gendered practices of childrearing. On the contrary, it highlights the need for the provision of additional support to families during the transitional phase. Thus, the hospital representatives' appeal to children's emotional comfort during medical procedures may be factually accurate without legitimizing the exclusion of fathers. (In many cases, of course, such appeal will be misleading: that is, in cases when the father *is* the primary caregiver of the child.) Instead, institutions may choose to take extra steps to attend to the children's emotional comfort if this is what is needed to enable fathers to support their children during hospitalization. For instance, hospitals could allocate more time to the treatment of children accompanied by fathers and give fathers psychological support in addressing the children's emotional needs. Current expectations and policies such as the ones discussed here presuppose that it is mothers or even women in general who are or should be children's primary carers. This not only discourages or altogether prevents fathers from taking care of their children when children also have a mother, but also sees relatives who may be less involved in children's lives as more appropriate carers than fathers. It, thus, effectively denies fathers' status as their children's carers.

The transition from gender-traditional to gender-egalitarian practices of childrearing often requires additional effort and resources in order to prevent the costs of this transition from falling on children. Critics may worry, first, that regulations meant to facilitate fathers' function as caregivers to their children constitute illegitimate interference within the privacy of the family. Second, they may see the spending of additional resources as an unfair use of public money. Both worries should be easy to dispel by appeal to children's interests. The aim of the state in enacting more progressive gender policies would not be to encourage a particular (gender-egalitarian) conception of the good on adults. It is, instead, to protect and foster the father–child relationship and effectively recognize fathers as well as mothers as caring parents.

In the petition mentioned earlier in this case study, parents complained that children's emotional comfort was clearly not what had motivated decisions to separate children from their parents in hospital wards: hospital practices had included restriction of movement and forcing treatment upon unwilling, distressed children. According to the parents, such practices have caused significant distress to their children, in addition to the distress of having been separated from their parents. Furthermore, a survey suggested that parents themselves, both mothers and fathers, do not align with the hospitals' policies to not allow fathers to stay in the hospital with their children, but instead deem them discriminatory and against the interests of both parents and children (Atudorei and Mardache 2012).

Legislative changes facilitating gender-egalitarian childrearing challenge current practices and expectations from fathers in Romania. At the same time, the nature of the relationship between patients, their families, and healthcare professionals is changing, and this leads to renegotiations and redefinitions of what is acceptable in a healthcare setting (Munthe et al. 2012). New laws often conflict both with existing practices and with people's expectations. Even when social expectations change, institutional practices may take their time and require further nudges before they adjust. In turn, these conflicts trigger processes that require the questioning and ultimately the abandoning of widespread gendered practices in childcare. These are constrained by the changing regulations as well as changing norms and expectations in the general population.

NOTES

1. The ways in which states choose to implement a preference for supporting co-parenting may raise their own set of issues. See, e.g., Bruno (2016) for an analysis of the consequences of the Swedish state's involvement in families separated by intrafamilial violence.
2. "(1) After the divorce, parental authority is shared by both parents, except when the court decides otherwise" (Art. 397) and "(1) In the absence of agreement between parents or if this is contrary to the superior interest of the child, at the time of the pronouncement of the divorce decision, the court establishes the child's residence at the parent with whom she has lived stably. (2) If the child has lived with both parents before the divorce, the court will establish the child's residence at one of the parents, keeping account of the child's superior interest" (Art. 400) (our translation).
3. The Council lacks the authority to enforce its decisions beyond issuing fines against individuals or other entities that are found to have discriminated.

REFERENCES

ActiveWatch, World Class. 2014. "Reguli Discriminatorii de Acces la Vestiar," November 19, 2014. activewatch.ro/ro/antidiscriminare/evenimente-si-activitati/world-class-reguli-discriminatorii-de-acces-la-vestiar.

Agerpres.ro, Ministerul Sanatatii. 2016. "Internarea copiilor mai mici de 14 ani, impreuna cu Unul Dintre Parinti, Este un Drept," May 10, 2016. agerpres.ro/sanatate/2016/05/10/ministerul-sanatatii-internarea-copiilor-mai-mici-de-14-ani-impreuna-cu-unul-dintre-parinti-este-un-drept-15-12-06.

Atudorei, Ioana, and Andreea Mardache. 2012. "Institutional Discrimination in Pediatric Hospitals." *Bulletin of the Transylvania University of Brasov* 5 (54) 2: 119–24.

Brighouse, Harry, and Adam Swift. 2014. *Family Values: The Ethics of Parent–Child Relationships*. Princeton, NJ: Princeton University Press.

Bruno, Linnéa. 2016. *Ofridstid. Fäders våld, staten och den separerade familjen*. Uppsala: Uppsala Universitet.

Collier, Richard, and Sally Sheldon. 2008. *Fragmenting Fatherhood: A Socio-Legal Study*. Oxford: Hart Publishing.

Curtea de Apel Bucuresti 2009 Sentinta Civila nr. 4180.

CNCD, Hotărirea nr. 649/04.12.2008.

Gheauş, Anca, and Ingrid Robeyns. 2011. "Equality-Promoting Parental Leave." *Journal of Social Philosophy* 42(2): 173–91.

Lindemann Nelson, Hilde, and James Lindemann Nelson. 1995. *The Patient in the Family: An Ethics of Medicine and Families*. New York: Routledge.

Monitorul Oficial no. 511, of July 24, 2009. www.dreptonline.ro/legislatie/codul_civil_republicat_2011_noul_cod_civil.php

Munthe, Christian, Lars Sandman, and Daniela Cutas. 2012. "Person Centred Care and Shared Decision Making: Implications for Ethics, Public Health and Research." *Health Care Analysis* 20(3): 231–49.

Ordin. 1284/2012. "Privind Reglamentarea Programului de Vizite al Apartinatorilor Pacientilor Internati in Unitatile Sanitare Publice." dreptonline.ro/legislatie/ordin_1284_2012_programul_de_vizite_apartinatori_pacienti_internati_unitati_sanitare_publice.php.

Parkinson, Patrick. 2011. *Family Law and the Indissolubility of Parenthood*. Cambridge: Cambridge University Press.

Parkinson, Patrick. 2006. "Fanily Law and the Indissolubility of Parenthood." *Family Law Quarterly* 40(2): 237–80.

Family Caregiving as a Problematic Category

JACQUELINE CHIN

Seventy-five-year-old Philomena Loh has been discharged from the hospital after two weeks, following an admission through the Accident and Emergency department for a stroke that has caused weakness in the left side of her body, including contractures in her left leg causing her knee to stiffen and stay bent. Philomena is otherwise mentally alert and her speech and swallowing reflexes have been unaffected. The hospital's discharge planning process involved helping Philomena's husband, Tom, 76, to prepare their home, a two-bedroom Housing and Development Board (HDB) apartment, for Philomena's return, including purchasing a wheelchair, installing ramps for wheelchair accessibility and a hospital bed for the ground-floor guest room, and hiring a foreign domestic worker, a 35-year-old Indonesian woman named Hana, through a special state-subsidized program for helping families to care for frail elderly relatives at home. Their daughter Stephanie, a television reporter, helped Tom and Philomena with the expenses for home remodeling and is paying Hana's salary, but work pressures make it hard for her to make regular visits to her parents. Philomena is relieved to return home and appreciates the effort that Tom and their daughter have made to provide for her care in her own home.

A week into her new job, Hana is having a difficult time. Intensely private, Philomena will not allow Hana to give her baths or dress her. Tom, who is exhausted, would like Hana to help Philomena with exercises to stretch her contracted knee, but Hana is disturbed by Philomena's screams from the pain of physiotherapy and would give up after a few weak attempts. Hana is distressed by Tom's anger at her seeming "incompetence" and inability to assist him with Philomena's needs, and by Philomena's rejection of her help. Hana is determined to telephone her agency on her next day off to seek a new placement, but before she does, Tom falls, suffers a brain hemorrhage, and is admitted to the hospital. Both Stephanie and Hana are filled with guilt and a deep sense of failure. Stephanie feels that perhaps her job is preventing her from attending more closely to her parents' needs. Hana feels disappointment and failure after having high hopes of securing work in Singapore that would pay her a better wage than her previous job as a shop assistant in Indonesia.

I. FAMILY CAREGIVING

This is a composite case description developed from interviews and workshop discussions (from July 2015 to February 2016) conducted by the author with health and social care workers grappling with Singapore's growing chronic disease burden. The project's purpose was to produce realistic case studies for a web-based, open access educational resource for teaching and learning bioethics. Interviews were first conducted with twenty-one aging and health policy experts, geriatricians, palliative care doctors, professionals in home care, and center-based and nursing home institutions on care transition issues. Group interviews were held during nine onsite visits (a nursing home, multiservice daycare center, rehabilitation center, hospital transition care service, geriatric ward for dementia care, dementia daycare center, group care home, community care hub at a psychiatric hospital, and the national care coordination agency). Five piloting workshops were conducted for reality testing of cases and to identify key issues to be included in ethics commentaries.

The present case focuses on (a) a typical household with a typical housing arrangement in Singapore, the HDB flat; (b) a care plan consistent with healthcare staffing policies for an aging population, which relies heavily on foreign domestic workers to support frail older people with dependency for activities of daily living at home when family caregivers have left home or are in the workforce; (c) a common age-related chronic condition and its particular care requirements; (d) care at home that typifies "aging in place" in accordance with healthcare planning policy.

In many aging societies, family caregiving is lauded as the ideal means of supporting "aging in place" (Wiles et al. 2012), but what is the category of "family caregiving" and how has it acquired its meaning and currency? In aging societies, care by families typically means keeping frail older people living in family homes, with appropriate services in place. In societies (like Singapore) with a significant "sandwich generation" where adult children take responsibility for parental care while juggling care of their own children and sometimes paid employment, the stress on working adults often means that heavier responsibilities for care of the frail elder fall upon spouses, who are themselves aging and growing frail. In this case, as in many other parts of the industrialized world, a live-in domestic worker is seen as a normal component of family caregiving (Eckenwiler 2012, 28). The presence of an extra pair of eyes and hands in the household to help with caring for a frail family member is reassuring from the perspective of hospital discharge planners and the aged spouse on whom primary caregiving has fallen.

This ideal of family caregiving needs reflective critique. In this commentary, family caregiving within the context of a health policy supporting "aging in place" for seriously ill seniors is problematized as a practice that reveals interstitial spaces (drawn from Vreugdenhil's research [2014]) in which complex goods and relationships are negotiated.

II. THE SOCIAL DISTRIBUTION OF CARE RESPONSIBILITY TO THE FAMILY

Recent research on family caregiving has cast a critical eye on social policies such as "aging in place" (Vreugdenhil 2014). While popular with older citizens and governments, these policies are known to redistribute care responsibilities that exact a toll on the overwhelming majority of family caregivers. Some of this research has yielded conceptually rich analyses of family caregiver experiences, demonstrating how caregivers (particularly adult women of the "sandwich generation") negotiate the "interstitial spaces" between individual needs/aspirations and caregiving roles (Eckenwiler 2012, 28). Those who choose (or feel no choice but) to take on family caregiving responsibilities must constantly juggle the mixed goods of close involvement with parents, children, and friends; self-care; and life and career advancement. These practices of self-conceptualization, distinctly gendered and particularly affecting women, are shaped by the framework of aging policies that set out the distribution of care work and care responsibilities according to an implicit value grid that puts at risk the family caregiver's health, quality of life, and financial adequacy. Hence, this research shows how social, cultural, and economic factors increase the complexity of questions about boundaries of responsibility for the individuals involved in family caregiving.

Critics of the aging-in-place principle have argued that the policies that grew out of those values focused on saving the state money, and expanding formal care services to afford more choice for the elderly, but have neglected to consider what serious choices are available to family caregivers. Whether social policies include options for family caregivers to refuse or limit caregiving roles and expectations (without penalty), and whether current "good employer" norms merely tolerate employees' caregiving are questions that have surfaced in this critical literature. One recent argument, leapfrogging over paid family leave and wages for housework, is the "caregiverist agenda," a call for a radical form of flexible work–life balancing that seeks to enable men and women to reorder the chronology of life, negotiating career and caregiving years over a longer lifespan, without penalty (Shulevitz 2016).

In some societies, "familialist" state ideologies may add the dimension of filial obligation as a further means of reinforcing norms of family caregiving. In Singapore, the law requires reasonable levels of financial support to be provided by children for parents who have no means of supporting themselves. The legislation, named the Maintenance of Parents Act to give explicit emphasis to the materialistic expression of filial piety, works through providing a means for a parent to lodge a complaint against a child for not providing financial support (Ministry of Social and Family Development 2015). By saying nothing about what counts as reasonable support (and whether other forms of support can replace the financial) or specifying which children are required to provide it, it leaves unaddressed many questions about fair distribution of filial duties among siblings. In attempting to prescribe boundaries and the scope of family caregiving responsibility, the law in meting out judgment cannot escape from engaging in a reflective task of understanding how responsibilities are negotiated within families and by individuals.

III. CONSCRIPTS TO "FAMILY CAREGIVING"

It is common in "familialist" cultures to reach for the easiest solution of transferring family care to low-wage live-in domestic workers. Humanitarian watchdog organizations within these cultures have raised awareness of the deeply unjust reality of the live-in worker's expected service. Many vulnerable young women from countries in the developing world have accepted unfair contracts which only vaguely specify job scope and description and expected working hours. In some countries, these contracts are not governed by employment law but are considered private arrangements between the foreign domestic worker and her local employer (Au-Yong 2016). Live-in domestic workers with poorly specified contracts often find themselves responsible for eldercare, childcare, meal preparation, housework, and the night shift to boot. The absence of contractual boundaries may well reflect a misrecognition of the domestic worker as "one of the family." There is no doubt that the paid worker in the home is inextricably a part of the family that depends on her, and on whom she depends for her orientation to the family's needs and rules of engagement. But this relationship and its proper regulation is wanting in countless cases like this.

Workers like Hana incur large risks when they undertake eldercare work in foreign homes with no proper training to do the job. They are often saddled with debt from loans taken to pay for their passage and transfer fees required by domestic worker agencies, sums that could take close to a year's wages to pay depending on how exploitative the situation is. If Hana is sent home in the event that she fails to secure a transfer to work in another household in Singapore, she could well bring long-term hardship and shame to her own family on her return to Indonesia as she struggles with this debt.

IV. FAULT LINES

This case also shows how the fault lines in family caregiving unravel in discharge planning for families with elders who grow frail. The caregiver spouse finds reassurance in the constant presence of a live-in helper, but this assurance turns out to be false. Tom's family home is not like the household Tom probably grew up in, where "amahs" (house servants belonging to sworn sisterhoods based in the Chinatowns of receiving cities like Singapore, Hong Kong, or San Francisco) lived as a part of the larger extended family for whom they worked. The migrant domestic worker situation has changed. Today's foreign domestic workers, like the amahs of the last generation, hail from traditional communities in which domestic servants have a quasi-family status within the household. However, receiving industrialized societies have changed the way in which the status of the domestic worker is configured within modern households, which have become nuclear household units, and "closeness" is a tightly guarded privilege reserved for the family unit of parents and children (Bradshaw 2014). In this household, we learn that Hana is "non-family" in spheres of privacy, such as bodily privacy or spaces of private suffering. Hana's plan to seek a transfer of employment is the common result. This case also shows that relationality (who counts as family and who does not) is a concept that must be situated in understandings of social change.

An ailing spouse, himself needing care, has succumbed to the physical stresses of home care and the new burdens of managing a crew of care providers—negotiating schedules, costs, and the quality and reliability of different services. The impression of autonomy in being able, as a consumer, to choose from a menu of professional care services belies the loss of independence faced by older persons like Tom and Philomena. The loss of past communities of care which offered older persons the freedom to choose to go to family or friends alike for assistance, and their replacement by nuclearized household units in which caregiving is shared by a very small number, can shatter the family peace if long-term care capacity is meager and provision of medical, social, personal, supportive, and residential needs is fragmented and costly for families. Families who are sensitive to costs or who shun the indignities of low-quality long-term care services for a loved one can hardly avoid taking on work that they are ill equipped and untrained to perform at home. Not uncommonly, the result is tragic, as has happened in the case of Tom, Philomena, Stephanie, and Hana. If family caregiving as described in this case study is seen as the gold standard of aging in place, opportunities may be missed for remodeling communities to enhance the independence and self-determination of persons growing old, and to open up spaces wider than the existing "interstitial" ones for their informal and paid caregivers.

V. SUMMARY

I have described what is well documented about present policies and practices of "family caregiving": they entail unjust distributions of care responsibility within and among countries and cause harm to those implicated in these structures. That said, families are likely to continue to be the indispensable and primary providers of long-term care for older people. Care is itself an undisputed foundation of any form of social life. Discussing the story of Philomena and her informal caregivers gives the outline of a challenging terrain and may help to chart a course for radical reconfiguration of social, material, and policy values that would enable caregivers to make nonpunitive, self-endorsed decisions across space (with more choices of sites of care) and over time (choosing the time for career development and the time for family caregiving) that honor and acknowledge real needs and actual capabilities.

REFERENCES

Au-Yong, Rachel. 2016. "Maids: Essential, or a Luxury?" *The Straits Times*, June 5. http://www.straitstimes.com/singapore/maids-essential-or-a-luxury, accessed July 5, 2016.

Bradshaw, Peter. 2014. "Ilo Ilo Review—Novelistic Singaporean Debut by Anthony Chen." *The Guardian*, May 1. https://www.theguardian.com/film/2014/may/01/ilo-ilo-review, accessed October 28, 2017.

Eckenwiler, Lisa A. 2012. *Long-Term Care, Globalization, and Justice*. Baltimore: Johns Hopkins University Press.

Ministry of Social and Family Development. 2015. *Report on Ageing Families in Singapore*. https://app.msf.gov.sg/Portals/0/Summary/research/FDG/Ageing%20Families%20Report%20Insight%20Series%2020151124.pdf, accessed July 5, 2016.

Shulevitz, Judith. 2016. "How to Fix Feminism." *New York Times*, June 10, 2016. http://www.nytimes.com/2016/06/12/opinion/sunday/how-to-fix-feminism.html?_r=0, accessed July 5, 2016.

Vreugdenhil, Anthea. 2014. "'Ageing-in-Place': Frontline Experiences of Intergenerational Family Carers of People with Dementia." *Health Sociology Review* 23(1): 43–52.

Wiles, Janine, Annette Leibing, Nancy Guberman, Jeanne Reeve, and Ruth E. S. Allen. 2012. "The Meaning of 'Aging in Place' to Older People." *Gerontologist* 52(3): 357–66.

Chapter 4

Healthcare Decisions

ULRIK KIHLBOM AND CHRISTIAN MUNTHE

Healthcare decisions about investigation, diagnosis, and treatment (including decisions not to apply measures, or to stop applying ongoing ones) may involve, engage, or affect family relations and family members of a patient in a variety of ways. This complicates the assessment of how options affect patients, and may furthermore elicit independent effects on professionals through expected actions of family members. Moreover, due to the close and intimate nature of the family relationships we are discussing here, *considerations* about such aspects may concern clinical professionals, patients, and family members independently of how they *actually* manifest themselves in terms of effects on length and quality of life, autonomy, and so on. In particular, decisions can be expected both to be influenced by and to affect family members' conceptions of mutual responsibilities making up the basic moral web of families, as pictured in Chapter 1 of this volume.

Irrespective of how family responsibilities are allocated or what legal requirements around medical decision making are in place in different particular situations, healthcare professionals are almost always expected to play an important role in the decision-making process. The aim of this chapter is to outline how different relational aspects of families may ground obligations on behalf of healthcare professionals toward patients and their families in the processes of decision making within healthcare.

To initiate painting this picture, we start from the core idea within person-centered care that patients' general life situation, experiences, values, and wants are substantial topics of concern in a process of shared decision making (Luxford 2010; Munthe et al. 2012; Sandman and Munthe 2010). Many have observed that, since most people have families, this will in practice force care to become more relation- or family-centered (Committee on Hospital Care and Institute for Patient- and Family-Centered Care 2012; Goodrich 2009; Ells et al. 2011; Luxford et al. 2010; Mead and Bower 2000; Munthe et al. 2012; Van Royen et al. 2010). The basic perspective of this book supports that observation and enriches it in several ways. One conclusion is that if the envisioned new decision-making paradigms are to be minimally functional, professionals' stances need to involve complex schemes of including people closely related to patients, who will have to be recognized as legitimate stakeholders and partners in, as well as resources for, clinical care.

We will briefly outline different aspects of family relations and then describe the normative implications these have for healthcare professionals in relation to healthcare decision making. This overview is complemented by an example which illustrates some of the complexities involved, linking to observations of ethical, moral, and psychological complications of clinical care of children and adolescents, made concrete by the context of care for diabetes type 1.

I. RELATIONAL ASPECTS OF PERSON CENTEREDNESS AND SHARED DECISION MAKING: A GENERAL OUTLINE

The relational aspects of person centeredness and shared decision making actualize a number of dimensions of relevance for ethical theory as well as for clinical practice. These will here be outlined briefly before some selected aspects are highlighted.

The Demarcation Between Patient Interests and the Interests of Others.

This is something noted already in ordinary clinical experience by many professionals, especially in areas where closely related persons usually are present in the care situation, such as obstetric and neonatal care, or terminal care of elderly persons. Family interests may upset, compete with, or complicate attending to the interests of the patient in clinical decision making. However, having person centeredness and shared decision making be influenced by familial relationships of whatever type seems to undermine the otherwise traditional notion in clinical ethics and practice for such situations, which is to always give the patient's best interests priority, and to potentially only include family members as *co-patients*, or legitimate concerned parties. First, most patients will include among their interests many concerns about their family members. Second, family members' interests and concerns may often go far beyond whatever biomedically defined health problem the patient has. Third, due to these factors, when healthcare concerns are widened to include more general aspects of patients' lives, the main basis for not considering effects of family members disappears. Fourth, this implies that healthcare decision making also needs to consider potential effects on core family goods, such as established patterns of (perceived) relations of responsibility, strong emotional dependencies, and attached bases of security and safety. This issue is explicitly formulated as a main challenge to family-centered care of children in the case study by Herlitz and Munthe in this chapter.

The Allocation of Professional, Patient, and Family Responsibilities.

This issue too is well known by healthcare professionals, especially those where the active assistance of family members is vital for the performance of care (often outpatient self-care); again, the cases of children and incapacitated elderly persons provide ample illustration. Emphasis on the relational aspects of person centeredness and shared decision making would here seem to highlight the idea of family members as *co-carers* (rather than co-patients), as the family situation of a patient will include considerations entering such clinical decision making by family members. This leads to issues of what responsibilities family members can and should be given or even required to provide and under what conditions. Such matters become especially complex in view of the understanding of families as webs of responsibility—that is, closely knit social units that already contain established perceptions of mutual responsibilities across a wide collection of areas; few of them may relate immediately to healthcare, but all of them may influence the potential consequences of chosen care measures. Consider, for instance, the case of a patient who requests important surgery, for which nonsmoking is a requirement, but whose partner is a heavy smoker. In the case study by Herlitz and Munthe, this aspect is highlighted, as it points to how family members will influence adolescent diabetes care performance, no matter what degree of their involvement in clinical decision making is chosen by professionals.

II. THE FAMILY AS A RESOURCE FOR CLINICAL ASSESSMENT AND DECISIONS

The indicated widened scope of clinical considerations means that the family becomes a possible positive resource for clinical decision

making in a number of ways, something the Herlitz and Munthe
case study exemplifies in the context of pediatrics. In this context,
family members are viewed as individuals who may contribute relevant information and offer support services to enable new caring
options. But the family is also seen as a social unit, which may provide what seems akin to the public goods produced by organized
societies that are important to the care, such as feelings of belonging,
security, acceptance, and closure in the face of a seriously impaired
or changed life situation. Of course, in the traditional pragmatics
of clinical practice, these aspects may be present to the extent that
practitioners spot them and find reason to take them into account,
but it is not a theme that is systematically applied or included in
guidelines for good clinical care. In some specific areas involving
gathering of biomedically relevant information, this aspect has been
openly and more systematically addressed—for example, in the case
of communicable disease or genetic testing. However, most of this
landscape of the family as a clinical resource seems to be passed over
in silence or actively avoided in the literature on the ethics of clinical
decision making.

III. THE FAMILY AS A THREAT
TO SUCCESSFUL CLINICAL DECISION
MAKING AND CARE

Just as the family of patients may be a resource for care and decision
making, so too can it be a threat to it. The widened scope for having the interests of family members and the family as a psychosocial
unit enter clinical decision making created by person centeredness
and shared decision making creates a much more far-reaching palette
of scenarios and aspects to consider. Again, the case study of adolescent diabetes care raises several examples of this. First, if the good

of family members and of families needs attention in the assessment of clinical options, this assessment may become impractical and too complex to be handled well by health professionals. Second, stark conflicts may appear between what a health professional considers the responsible thing to do and what is desired either by the patient (out of family concerns) or by family members affected by the situation, and the relational aspect makes it less obvious how such conflicts should be analyzed. Third, incapacities, structures, or wants not of the patient but of the patient's family may block otherwise available care strategies requiring family collaboration, and it is unclear how far health professionals may venture to change such situations, or even force changes.

A main observation regarding these four central areas is that they seem to require health professionals to systematically address issues for which they are not normally trained. Moreover, standard principles in clinical bioethical and healthcare ethical frameworks provide scant support, as they usually rest on the assumption that the areas we describe are unusual exceptions rather than the quotidian ones they become if a family-centered approach to person centeredness and shared decision making is adopted in earnest.

IV. RELATIONAL NORMATIVITY AND PATIENT INTERESTS

So far, we have touched on solely empirical and practical complications of taking seriously a family-centered approach to care. These all have to do with the multiplication of interests, parties, and stakes that follow if the conception of a family as a moral web of responsibilities that may contain goods of its own is applied to notions of person centeredness and shared decision making. However, the emphasis on relational aspects of patients' autonomy and goods prominent in this book also raises underlying conceptual concerns regarding the very notion of *patient interest*.

One aspect of this notion that needs to be considered links to the inherently normative nature of family relations. Such relations are in part constituted by responsibilities, commitments, and entitlements that hold between those standing in a familial relationship to each other, even though it might be unclear or controversial exactly which those are. A sign of this normativity is the way in which people may justify actions toward family members, well known, for example, in the case of organ donation discussed in the case study by Scully in this chapter. Suppose that Annie's brother Stewart has an end state renal disease and that he is in need of a kidney. He asks Annie, who is a biologically suitable donor partly because they are siblings, to consider a donation, and she agrees to donate one of her kidneys. According to her, this is what she ought to do, and if someone were to ask her why, it would make perfect sense for Annie to reply: "He is my brother." That is, she would express a moral commitment to and responsibility for Stewart in virtue of their familial relationship, and this commitment constitutes her reason for donating a kidney to him. Now, certainly, part of this story is about the pragmatics of biological relatedness that makes Annie a particularly fitting donor for Stewart, but this is not all of it. Without the mentioned commitments and recognized responsibilities, Annie would have no more reason to donate a kidney to Stewart than to any other person she would biologically match in a similar way, and it is the presence of these normative relations which make Annie and Stewart *family* in the sense applied in the present volume. None of this is to say that these normative relations need to be ethically sound or that perceptions of such responsibilities cannot be reasonably disputed.

When we regard the relations defining families as normative, the notion of *the patient's interest* becomes less sharply demarcated than commonly assumed in healthcare and related ethics. One context in which this difficulty of separating a patient's interests from the interests of his or her family and its members may surface when the patient forms his or her notions of what care to prefer out of consideration of perceived family interests. Think of an elderly patient with his reasoning capacities intact and in the end of his life, who after some years at a nursing home requests an ongoing life-sustaining treatment to stop because he wishes to relieve his children from the burden of worrying about him and visiting him on an almost daily basis. Or, similarly but the other way around, the patient prefers further life-sustaining treatment for his children's sake, although he would otherwise just as well have it discontinued. In such cases, we may, of course, worry about manipulation or undue emotional pressure, say, due to content or discontent expressed by the children. We might also, on a more societal level, be concerned about the causes of such a burden, if it arises out of poor public support or from scant value given to older lives. However, these types of considerations may be made quite regardless of that. It is not in any way strange if the man wants to die for his children's sake, although the children harbor no such wish, and he may want to survive for their sake, although they would prefer him to die.

Either way, these kinds of considerations are bound to cause some uneasiness among healthcare professionals caring for a person in such a situation, as well as some bewilderment by ethicists who are supposed to assist them—and rightly so. As indicated, there are good reasons to be cautious and attentive when motivations such as these are at play. Patients in the end of life are often vulnerable to manipulation and susceptible to conditions such as depression, which may cause irrational self-disregard. However, other-regarding motivations are not as such excluded from properly belonging to the patient's *own* interests. A patient, or any person for that matter, may take her other-regarding concerns to trump her self-regarding ones without losing the ownership, as it were, of those interests. We will in the next section return to the question of how the distinction between the interests of person and family can be understood and the implication for family-centered decision making. But before that, we make one final point about the relational normativity brought to the fore of a family-centered approach to clinical decision making.

V. BOUNDARY PROBLEMS

When acting toward a family member we may find ourselves in situations that may be experienced as no-choice situations, where our place in the web of family responsibilities creates a kind of moral necessity. The case of Annie in the case study by Scully may exemplify this. Her perception of the situation may well be that to donate her kidney is something she *must* do—there "really" is no other option. This type of response is probably quite common whenever an important healthcare measure requires the participation or assistance of family members; they tend to agree to such a role immediately, without much deliberation, and are quick to embed this new role into their daily life, as when a partner helps with mobility and exercise in the home, remembers medication and diet, or tends to simpler care tasks (such as changing bandages). In practical action, they thereby accept such roles, and certainly do not object to it, but neither do they ever actively endorse it or consciously make a resolution to take it up. Rather, they are morally compelled by their family responsibilities.

With a single-minded application of a traditional conception of freedom to such a response pattern, one may well end up with the conclusion that people thus responding to a perceived moral necessity of family responsibilities are coerced by circumstances outside of their control. The lack of conscious choice due to moral pressure and the lack of perceived alternatives may be thought to support the idea that people in such circumstances therefore cannot be fully exercising their autonomy. On a standard view, freedom is roughly a matter of having the power to act otherwise than what one in fact does, and a very common notion is that such power presupposes that the subject of the freedom believes it to be in place—what is sometimes referred to as the *epistemic condition* of freedom and responsibility (Eshleman 2014). However, when a person feels morally compelled, not able to see any real alternative in the sense here exemplified, the presence of such a belief may be doubted. And if that is the case, the acting parties in such situations cannot, by the standard formula of "ought implies can," be responsible for whatever moral valence befalls their actions.

However, this line of reasoning has been questioned, as in the case of organ donation between siblings (Crouch and Elliott 1999). The web of strong emotional ties between a sister who donates a vital organ, her brother who receives it, and their parents who thereby have the life of one of their children saved, cannot by itself undermine autonomy and moral responsibility. The notion of ruling ourselves in the way required for moral agency and responsibility must be compatible with having strong emotional and moral commitments to specific others, also in situations when they create a sense of having no choice besides acting on them. Simply put, if the possession of normative moral reasons presupposes freedom, this freedom cannot in turn exclude that people possess such reasons. At the same time, coercion and undue influences do occur within families and are then usually exercised through the web of emotional as well as moral relations that constitute them—emotional blackmail being a familiar example of a source of family members experiencing having no choice in a way that is obviously problematic from an autonomy standpoint. Thus, the challenge is to recognize that people who act out of strong concern for each other or their shared community may very well act just as freely as those who act out of a classic notion of self-interest, while simultaneously recognizing that such interpersonal concerns and sentiments may constitute risk factors for undue influence that may undermine autonomy and responsibility.

One influential way to account for these distinctions is to say that it is a matter of how *I*, as a subject or person, *relate to* my interests and commitments—how well they cohere with each other and other aspects of my view of myself and my life in the world. The immediate, strong motivation of normative reasons that originate from a subject and are endorsed by himself or herself and are experienced as a "must" has been coined *volitional necessity* (Frankfurt 1971). This type of experienced necessity is easy to imagine influencing a person like Annie, or any other possible donor to any sort of family member, to set aside what she would otherwise have wanted for her own sake (even to the point of silencing it altogether) when facing the vital need of her brother. We may assume that anyone in such circumstances acknowledges and accepts such a vividly experienced normative requirement: we *want* to do what we experience that we must do for the sake of those close to us. In this way, by endorsing our commitments and their motivational pull, our concerns for others can be said to be proper parts of our own interests. Thereby, we remain autonomous in the morally relevant sense also when, in light of such commitments, we have an experience of having to donate an organ or tissue to others (to take one instance), as long as we endorse the moral authority it exercises on us, and this holds even if we perceive no alternative and may thus be argued to fail, technically, the epistemic condition of moral responsibility.

Suppose that someone who is continuously assisting in the care of a partner, a child, a parent, a sibling, for reasons of the type just described starts to be less comfortable with the arrangement, even outright disliking it, yet continues to provide care out of the strong feelings of obligation. Would this person now act less autonomously, even be a victim of (inner) coercion? For the same reason as before, it seems plausible to deny such a suggestion, as deciding to act against personal desires for moral reasons is a part of our ordinary struggling with competing considerations, some of which are moral. This is not to deny that when the situation changes in this way, things begin to get morally more complicated. If starting to doubt whether the caring effort should continue, would it be acceptable for others to put pressure on us to continue, and insist on the moral reasons to care for family members? This, it seems, depends more on *why* caring for our family member has become less of a sure thing than on *how uncomfortable* or *how compelling* we find it to act on what we see as our moral duty.

Now, suppose that the very *commitment* to care for our close one gradually weakens over the years. This may occur in two ways. One is that we change our perception of the balance of reasons; we still embrace a commitment and experience a duty of care for our family member, but now find the cost to ourselves to be too high. The other is that we let go of our commitment to care for our family member; that is, we dislodge some of the nodes in the web of responsibility making us family in the first place. Other members of our family may then react by putting pressure on us to remain within what they see as an adequate balance of reasons and web of responsibilities, which we no longer subscribe to. Such pressure may then approach what is clearly undue influence, especially if it contains elements of threatening to withdraw personal and emotional contact and this has us go on with the caring against our own best judgment. This action will no longer be exercised from within our personal commitments but from external forces and fear of sanction.

However, even if no such obvious situation of compliance due to threat occurs, and even if a person very much embraces his or her relational commitments to family members, we may still find the situation ethically problematic. Again, the decisive thing seems to be what explains *why* a person entertains a commitment (or not), and what may worry us is that it may result from an oppressive or manipulative context, as in the case of religious or political sects, dysfunctional families, and so on. Whether a person is autonomous cannot merely be due to the internal coherence of a set of wants and commitments, as such sets may arise out of circumstances that bypass the emotional and cognitive mechanisms supposed to be involved in autonomous decision making, thus undermining autonomy even in the absence of outright threat or coercion.

At the same time, it may be argued that families contain such oppressive and manipulative structures much more often and strongly than usually acknowledged—for instance, regarding gender and age roles. Suppose that John needs a kidney and his younger wife, Emma, is a suitable donor. John is in his sixties and Emma has just turned forty, and they have a daughter of five who suffers from idiopathic nephrotic syndrome, indicating a risk of future renal problems. Suppose also that they are part of a typical patriarchal (paternalist, sexist, and ageist) family structure, where the expectation is that Emma, whatever hardships are implied, will stand by her man. When, in a private consultation with a nephrologist, Emma says that she wants to donate, the nephrologist is worried and points out that their daughter might need a kidney in the future. But Emma remains unmoved. She fully endorses the family's relational moral requirement to donate her kidney in order to be a loyal wife for better or for worse—even if that implies becoming less ready to care for her daughter in the future.

One way to try to pinpoint what in the explanation of Emma's commitment to her husband grounds a suspicion of undue influence is to identify her apparent unresponsiveness to reason. To be autonomous one must arguably have a capacity to navigate among different norms and values and to somehow respond to them—this is a part of the cognitive and emotional apparatus indicated earlier in the chapter. But for such responsiveness to be attainable to people who perceive themselves as having responsibilities toward one another, they have to mutually acknowledge and respect that each may have reason to reconceive these responsibilities; the relational structure has to make room for its web of responsibilities to change. If John and the rest of Emma's social environment does not allow for this, her values may not properly be her own and her autonomy may be impaired due to her relational environment's blocking her access to what she would otherwise recognize as important reasons. Coercion and undue influence may, hence, be structurally embedded in some common responsibility webs making up families, and constantly have some of its members suffer persistent loss of autonomy regarding certain choices they make out of relational concern. The challenge is to pinpoint when this is the case and when it is not.

VI. THE ETHICS OF THE FAMILY AS CO-CARER

As indicated, besides being active parties in decision making, or being part of a context that requires advanced attention in clinical decision making, family centeredness opens considerable space for a patient's family to be included not only as assistants (as in the case of organ donation) but as actual performers of care: *co-carers*. Again, this phenomenon has always been present in various forms of outpatient care, but the family-centered move creates more transparency around how this is done, a wider space for professionals to systematically consider family members as co-carers, and an implied shift of power and responsibility to family (besides the one toward patients implied by the person-centered approach), with regard, for example, to what they are prepared to accept in terms of work required, financial sacrifices, changes of internal family structures and traditions, accountability for the outcome of care, and so on. This also means that care solutions where the family and its members are made co-carers become both possible and necessary to assess more systematically from an ethical standpoint. In Chapter 5, relevant issues of social justice and responsibility will be addressed. Here, we will mention four more immediate ethical aspects of this.

First, the more of a co-carer the family becomes, the more critical becomes the issue of how well prepared it and its members are to take on that responsibility, and what responsibility health professionals have to facilitate or guarantee that requirements in this area are met. This has been highlighted as a central ethical issue of person-centered care and shared decision making with regard to patients (Munthe et al., 2012). Family co-carers in this context are expected to independently perform continuous clinical assessment, decision making, and execution of measures, but at the same time lack the overall specialist knowledge and skills of a trained and experienced health professional. At the same time, the person-centered shift opens up room for considering solutions and plans where family is included as co-carer. Which arrangements are defensible and why, and what responsibility for such arrangements and their outcomes befall family and health professionals respectively? It makes sense to claim that if health professionals actively pursue family involvement that expands the co-caring role, they also have a responsibility to secure the quality of this delegation of decision making and service. But to what extent? And to what extent is the ethics of such allocations of responsibility for co-caring dependent on the extent to which they arise at the behest of the patient and the family themselves?

The next two aspects both link to the assumption that family relationships involve particular intimacy, implying close and strong emotional relatedness, knowledge about personal details, shared assumptions about what is expected and of value in the family situation, and so on. This feature of a patient's family has an immediate instrumental importance in that it may be mobilized for both good and bad, as elaborated in earlier sections of the chapter. The intimacy may, of course, be a great resource that can improve care, and in some respects makes the co-care of family superior to that delivered by an occasionally visiting health professional. However, the same intimacy may also serve to harm patients, since a role as co-carer may make family members cross boundaries they should not cross, as well as reinforce abusive or oppressive family structures already in place. It may even provide new tools for family members to exploit the intimacy for getting at each other or upset internal relationship structures to the detriment of patients. Second, the intimacy also connects to the mentioned difficulty of keeping apart the interests of patients and of the family (and its members). Depending on how co-caring of family members is organized, it may give more or less room for patient interests flowing out of internal family relationships, such as a will to avoid burdening one's intimates, or the opposite tendency of making those close to oneself increasingly dependent on a continued co-caring relationship.

The final aspect we want to highlight comes out of the idea of families producing special relational goods (or evils) accessible to family members, akin to the public goods usually assumed to be produced by organized societies. Many of these seem to link to the way in which families assemble themselves into an informal social organization, where members unassumingly occupy and play specific roles to co-produce goods available to all family members to make life valuable and meaningful (or the opposite)—for example, senses of belonging, safety, and identity (or lack of such). The role as co-carer in organized healthcare efforts, however, seems to pull out of and break these qualities of the typical family web of relationships, as the *informal* relations are now transformed and linked to a formally institutionalized external web of norms, standards, and evaluators (the health professionals, who deliver the verdict on how the care is proceeding). The question is what this means for the family's internal production of relational goods and how that is to be factored into the ethical assessment of various ways in which family can be made co-carer in family-centered healthcare decision making.

VII. IMPLICATIONS FOR THE RESPONSIBILITIES OF HEALTHCARE PROFESSIONALS

In light of the different aspects we have outlined, we might now turn to the question of what normative expectations are reasonable to put on healthcare professionals in the context of healthcare decision making with patients and their families.

First, there is a process-oriented task to facilitate deliberation and decision making. Obviously, reaching decisions about medical treatment is a process rather than a single action or event. This means, at least, that there is a route to the decision that stretches over a period of time, and that this route includes a number of steps that leads to the decision—steps that involve smaller decisions, meetings, exchanging and processing information, reasoning, and so forth. Experienced clinicians often talk about the importance of creating a deliberative space when facing a serious clinical decision—to put the decision on hold while grounding it in different ways. Timewise, a deliberative space can in the clinical setting vary between minutes and months. Above the temporal aspect, there are conceptual, emotional, and discursive aspects of a deliberative space. Such a space may allow the parties to conceptualize the alternative actions, to reflect emotionally on the alternatives, and to discuss feelings and attitudes toward the decision. Properly articulated, such a space may also allow for relatives and close ones to take part in the deliberative process. We might think of decision processes in healthcare as involving a number of deliberative spaces, where each precedes a decision of varying magnitude. Deliberative spaces are no novelty, but there are reasons to stress that they are of our making, and that healthcare professionals are crucial in framing the decision process properly. It is, therefore, their responsibility to create or to foster deliberative spaces that allow a number of relational aspects to be brought to the forefront of the decision-making process. The extent to which healthcare professionals should be active or even authoritative in the deliberation is highly dependent upon contextual features of the patient, the family, the disease, the treatment, and so forth.

Among the relational aspects that need to be identified are, as we have indicated, shared interests—family interests. Without entering into in-depth issues of social ontology, we might state that these belong both to single individuals and to collectives. The sorting out of what interests are shared with others or more solely belong to an individual is an important deliberative task, central for both the patient–family constellation and healthcare professionals. If this is accomplished to a satisfactory degree, the identification of responsibilities is more easily addressed. For healthcare professionals, it will also be important to identify what emotional leverage close relations may equip family members with in cases of decision making. As we have described, undue influence and emotional coercion may go in different directions.

In summary, as well as respecting this sense of relational autonomy of the patient and family, healthcare professionals have a significant responsibility to promote it in the different ways indicated here.

REFERENCES

Committee on Hospital Care and Institute for Patient- and Family-Centered Care. 2012. "Patient- and Family-Centered Care and the Pediatrician's Role." *Pediatrics* 129(2): 394–404.

Crouch, Robert A., and Carl Elliot. 1999. "Moral Agency and the 'Family': The Case of Living Related Organ Transplantation." *Cambridge Quarterly of Healthcare Ethics* 8 (3): 275–87.

Ells, Carolyn, Matthew R. Hunt, and Jane Chambers-Evans. 2011. "Relational Autonomy as an Essential Component of Patient-Centered Care." *International Journal of Feminist Approaches to Bioethics* 4(2): 79–101.

Eshleman, Andrew. 2014. "Moral Responsibility." *Stanford Encyclopedia of Philosophy*, ed. Edward N. Zalta. http://plato.stanford.edu/archives/sum2014/entries/moral-responsibility/ (accessed August 10, 2016).

Frankfurt, Harry. 1971. "Freedom of the Will and the Concept of a Person." *Journal of Philosophy* 68(1): 5–20.

Goodrich, Joanna. 2009. "Exploring the Wide Range of Terminology Used to Describe Care That Is Patient-Centred." *Nursing Times* 105(20): 14–17.

Lindemann, Hilde. 2007. "Care in Families." In *Principles of Health Care Ethics*, ed. Richard E. Ashcroft, Angus Dawson, Heather Draper, and John R. McMillan, 351–56. Chichester, UK: Wiley.

Luxford, Karen, Donella Piper, Nicola Dunbar, and Naomi Poole. 2010. *Patient-Centred Care: Improving Quality and Safety by Focusing Care on Patients and Consumers*. Sydney: Australian Commission of Quality and Safety in Health Care.

Mead, Nicola, and Peter Bower. 2000. "Patient-Centeredness: A Conceptual Framework and Review of the Empirical Literature." *Social Science and Medicine* 51: 1087–110.

Munthe, Christian, Lars Sandman, and Daniella Cutas. 2012. "Person-Centred Care and Shared Decision-Making: Implications for Ethics, Public Health and Research." *Health Care Analysis* 20: 231–49.

Sandman, Lars, and Christian Munthe. 2010. "Shared Decision-Making, Paternalism and Patient Choice." *Health Care Analysis* 18: 60–84.

Van Royen, Paul, Martin Beyer, Patrick Chevallier, Sophia Eilat-Tsanani, Christos Lionis, Lieve Peremans, Imre Rurik, Jean Karl Soler, Inre Ejh Stoffers, Pinar Tosever, Mehmet Ungan, and Eva Hummers-Pradier. 2010. "The Research Agenda for General Practice/Family Medicine and Primary Health Care in Europe. Part 3. Results: Person-Centred Care, Comprehensive and Holistic Approach." *European Journal of General Practice* 16: 113–19.

Family Centeredness as Resource and Complication in Outpatient Care with Weak Adherence, Using Adolescent Diabetes Care as a Case in Point

ANDERS HERLITZ AND CHRISTIAN MUNTHE

Consider two clinical situations from pediatric diabetes care.[1] In both situations, an adolescent diabetes patient (P), her parent (PP), and a health professional (HP) are present:

Situation 1

HP: I see that your blood sugar value was a bit high here, between 12 and 14.

PP: Between 12 and 14, you say? That's bad, P! Haven't we spoken about this? It should be lower!

P: I know ...

HP: Do you know what a good value is?

PP: She does know, isn't that right, P?

P: Yes . . .

PP: You need to listen to what HP says here. Your health is at stake!

Situation 2

HP: I see that your blood sugar value was a bit high here, between 12 and 14.

P: Yeah . . .

PP: It was a stressful period for P. Many things were going on; you know how it can be to be a teenager.

HP: I know it can be tough, but you do know that you should try to keep the value lower?

P: Yes, I know.

PP: Maybe we can figure out a way to keep the blood value in shape also in stressful situations.

In the first situation, the parent does at least these three things: (1) showing off her own knowledge of the illness; (2) placing a heavy responsibility on the child; and (3) speaking for the child. In the second situation, the parent takes a different attitude by (1) helping the child by explaining the HP's observation; (2) initiating a search for creative solutions; and (3) letting the child speak first. In this brief report, we address how family members can play both a positive and a negative role in situations that require large amounts of outpatient care and point to some ethical questions that arise in relation to this.

Care for adolescent patients with type 1 diabetes is a recognized challenge, with known adherence problems in a context where home care, self-care, and day-to-day lifestyle adjustments are vital. The recommended care regimen often gives rise to conflicts with broader personal and social needs and desires, and in the case of weak adherence, negative spirals of undermined self-confidence and/or emotional denial may result, aggravating the situation (Boman et al. 2015; Delameter 2007; Diabetes Control and Complications Trial Study Group 1995; Herlitz et al. 2016). The need to adjust care to the specific situation is accepted within the pediatric diabetes professional community, accepting a commitment to person centeredness (Ekman et al. 2011; Luxford, et al. 2010), and alliance with the family is a critical part of this (Delameter 2007; Shields et al. 2006). Yet, as the two situations at the beginning of the chapter illustrate, families can be involved in different ways, and the issue of *how* to involve families and what ethical tensions that may actualize is largely unexplored.

Standard models of person and family centeredness tell us little about how to involve family members in care similar to that of diabetes. Typically, the models focus on trying to engage and educate patients and their family to decide and implement ready-made options, often in a hospital setting (Boman et al. 2015; Herlitz et al. 2016). These models are thus poorly equipped to address problems like diabetes that require self-care and lifestyle adjustment by patients with vulnerable decision-making capacities in a mostly outpatient context (Entwistle and Watt 2013; Naik et al. 2009). We have elsewhere proposed an alternative approach more attuned to such circumstances, aiming less for rational decision making in consultation meetings and more at empowering patients' long-term capacities to manage their condition at home (Herlitz et al. 2016).

This "counseling, self-care, adherence (CSA)" approach offers a look at the role that family can play to improve these types of care. We will illustrate how family members can assist in the care of teenagers with diabetes but that there are also serious risks actualized by such involvement. In particular, we will highlight ethical complications that arise when the role of a family member is changed from "parent" to "care provider."

I. THE CSA APPROACH

Successful treatment of illnesses that require substantial outpatient measures such as lifestyle adjustments and self-treatment actualizes decision making both inside the clinical setting and at home. Successful treatment relies on deliberative clinical decisions that require attention, focus, and time. Treatment success, however, relies mostly on day-to-day decisions, which are mostly intuitive, not involving much conscious attention or preceded by elaborate deliberation. For diabetes patients such decisions include eating and drinking, physical exercise, use of drugs, monitoring glucose levels, and adjusting daily activities. However, most of the attention of care targets only the first sort of deliberative decisions, falsely assuming that patients will automatically align their behavior to what was decided in clinical meetings with professionals. This is exemplified in both of the examples at the beginning of the chapter when the health professional raises the technical issue of blood sugar values. In reality, however, few individuals, and even fewer adolescents, work in that way. There is a significant difference between knowing what a good blood sugar value is and acting so that one attains a good blood sugar value.

The CSA approach is designed to address this challenge and identifies three general and transformable elements that influence how a patient's decisions at home align with treatment plans that were decided in clinical meetings but are supposed to be implemented by the patient on a day-to-day basis: (1) *internalization of care goals*, (2) *relevant perception of choice situations*, and (3) *empowering emotional feedback*.

Internalized goals are located within the wider framework of a person's goals and are therefore less likely to give rise to conflicts. A diabetic teen who decides, say, to exercise more will do better if she finds a way to internalize this goal within her wider framework of independently embraced interests. For example, if she is generally interested in competing and also generally interested in spending time in nature, she can try to develop an interest in some competitive outdoor sport. In this way, she will be more motivated to act in accordance with the care objective simply by pursuing the interests she already has. By raising the issue of how to find a way to have diabetes care objectives fit better with the stressful life of a teenager, the parent in the second situation can be seen as taking a step toward improving the internalization of the care goals.

A patient's perception will have an impact on her ability to implement it at home. Someone who spontaneously perceives cars as dangerous vehicles will be more careful when crossing a street. Likewise, a person with diabetes who perceives jam as an unhealthy condiment with high amounts of sugar will take this into account when deciding what to spread on her toast (to the extent that the care goal of avoiding sweet food has been internalized). By developing a way of seeing the world that categorizes choices in a way that is relevant from a diabetes care perspective, the patient can better align her care decisions with planned treatment goals. This aspect is completely overlooked in both of the situations at the beginning of the chapter, as the focus remains on the goal itself, not how its realization may be situated in the patient's daily life.

Finally, it is important to provide empowering emotional feedback to a person who has problems adhering to a care plan to build a sense of confidence that things can get better. For example, a person who is constantly reminded that she is failing to reach an idealized goal (say, a narrowly defined interval of HbA1c) is more likely to despair, develop an incapacitating self-image, and become less inclined to make new attempts. This is particularly relevant for adolescent, nonadherent patients with chronic conditions, who are in a stage of developing a more set adult identity. In the first example at the beginning of the chapter, the parent can be seen as providing destructive emotional feedback that threatens to undermine the young woman's future ability to do better.

II. FAMILY AND THE CSA APPROACH

Family plays an essential role in the CSA approach, as its key elements are at work at home. Family can contribute relevant information beyond what is offered by patients, as illustrated in the second situation. Parents, siblings, and close friends may all be able to make less biased assessments and see more clearly how a patient reacts to stress, peer pressure, disappointments, and so on. The presence of family members may serve to enhance the dialogue between caregivers and patients—for example, by relaxing conversation, by helping to focus the discussion on topics of relevance, or by raising important issues that patients or professionals neglect.

However, when the family of the patient is brought into the clinical conversation, so will all of its dysfunctions and tensions. For each potential benefit of involving family, there is therefore a risk. In the first situation the parent increases the tension, while in the second situation the parent relaxes it. Parents may hold false impressions of their children and misinform professionals, their presence might intimidate the child so that dialogue is prevented, or the parents' own interests and concerns may dominate meetings while relevant issues are neglected.

Whatever negative or positive results are achieved in clinical settings may be undermined when the patient leaves the protected environment of the clinic. Family members *will* influence the outcome of a CSA approach, no matter how much they are brought into or kept outside of clinical situations where care plans are decided. Family members provide resources to satisfy basic needs and to support child and adolescent development, and they influence the ways of being and thinking adopted by the young person. All of these factors contribute to the child's developing ability to handle care. Family members play a crucial role in patients' ability to internalize health goals and in how they perceive choice situations, and a family's emotional feedback can safely be assumed to be more influential than that of health professionals. Acting on caring impulses, however, they may easily adopt an ineffective nagging strategy instead of changing the patient's perception of everyday choices. Yet family may just as well counteract the destructive effects of, say, overly rigid health professionals by confirming the young person's feelings, making him or her feel safe, and providing emotional room for a more flexible view of how the care may be adapted. Rather than an "all or nothing" case, the issue is about how, and how much, to involve family.

III. ETHICAL CHALLENGES OF FAMILY-CENTERED CSA CARE

Concluding this brief case study, we will set out systematically what we take to be the chief *ethical* aspects of the family-related challenges mentioned.

A central challenge is for teams and professionals simply to be aware of these aspects. We have observed that while they may take on board the need to support patients' decision making at home, the ethical complications of family tend to be shunned as impossible to attend to, or as lying outside the clinic's organizational charter. Alas, this may make professionals less likely to address complications that they actually could do something about.

This difficulty may link to another one, namely that of possessing adequate competence to handle family-related challenges. This competence is, then, partly about *recognizing* significant ethical challenges in the clinical practice of family-centered care but also about *handling and responding* to these in an adequate way. Responding involves two elements: first, *being able to analyze the problems*, including expected disagreements, and, second, *implementing identified solutions* successfully. Both of these offer difficulties with an ethical twist, such as the presence in the professional training of adequate knowledge and skill, the composition and organization of the clinical team, and the institutional relationship between health and social care.

There are also core professional ethical issues, and we will mention two that we have found especially emergent in our studies of adolescent diabetes care. First, there is the question of how to allocate responsibilities. This is a complex issue when we consider just the patient and a professional; when the family aspect is considered, it becomes immensely more so, since the family already embodies a dense web of existing caring relations, where the interests of the patient are just one among many. In our material, we have observed how, apparently unwittingly, all responsibility is laid on the shoulders of a young patient while parents and clinicians ally in joint resentment and disappointment over his or her performance (Hartvigsson et al.), illustrated by the first situation at the beginning of the chapter.

Moreover, these family relations are often central to the core values and meaning that members of the family experience in and give to their personal lives. What does it mean for the continued existence of these values to blur the line, either intentionally or merely by recognizing its inevitability, between care provider and family member? Are we stuck with a painful, albeit necessary, tradeoff between preserving the values of family relations and improving health? And if so, what *is* the adequate tradeoff? Or are healthcare professionals licensed to intervene to change the inner relations of families for the sake of their patients' health? If so, how far does *that* license carry?[2]

NOTES

1. The cases emulate a number of concrete situations that we have observed in collaborative work with health professionals in this area.
2. Work on this chapter has been undertaken within the the projects *Comparability, Incommensurabilities, Value Conflicts and Priority Setting in the Health Care Sector*, funded by the Marie Curie International Postdoc Fellowship Program of the Swedish Research Council for Health, Working Life and Welfare (FORTE), contract no. 2014-2724; *Practices of Responsibility in Change*, funded by the Dutch Research Council (NWO); *Addressing Ethical Obstacles to Person Centered Care*, funded by FORTE and the Swedish Research Council (VR), contract no. 2014-4024; and the *Gothenburg Responsibility Project*, funded by VR, contract no. 2014-40.

REFERENCES

Boman, Å., M. Bohlin, M. Eklöf, G. Forsander, and M. Törner, 2015. "Conceptions of Diabetes and Diabetes Care Among Young People with Minority Background." *Qualitative Health Research* 25: 5–15.

Delamater A. M. 2007. "Psychological Care of Children and Adolescents with Diabetes." *Pediatric Diabetes* 8: 340–48.

Diabetes Control and Complications Trial Study Group 1995. "The Relationship of Glycaemic Exposure (HbA1c) to the Risk of Development and Progression of Retinopathy in the Diabetes Control and Complication Trial." *Diabetes* 44: 968–83.

Ekman, I., K. Swedberg, C. Taft, A. Lindseth, A. Norberg, A., E. Brink, and K. Stibrant Sunnerhagen. 2011. "Person-Centered Care: Ready for Prime Time." *European Journal of Cardiovascular Nursing* 10: 248–51.

Entwistle, V. A., and I. S. Watt. 2013. "Treating Patients as Persons: A Capabilities Approach to Support Delivery of Person-Centered Care." *American Journal of Bioethics* 13: 29–39.

Hartvigsson, T., G. Forsander, and C. Munthe. n.d. "Error Trawling and Fringe Decision Competence: Ethical Hazards in Monitoring and Addressing Patient Decision Capacity in Clinical Practice." Unpublished manuscript.

Herlitz, A., C. Munthe, M. Törner, and G. Forsander. 2016. "The Counseling, Self-Care, Adherence Approach to Person-Centered Care and Shared Decision-Making: Moral Psychology, Executive Autonomy and Ethics in Multidimensional Care Decisions." *Health Communications* 31(8): 964–73.

Luxford, K., D. Piper, N. Dunbar, and N. Poole. 2010. *Patient-Centred Care: Improving Quality and Safety by Focusing Care on Patients and Consumers*. Sydney: Australian Commission of Quality and Safety in Health Care.

Naik, A. D., C. B. Dyer, M. E. Kunik, and L. B. McCullough. 2009. "Patient Autonomy for the Management of Chronic Conditions: A Two-Component Reonceptualization." *American Journal of Bioethics* 9: 23–30.

Shields, Linda, Jan Pratt, and Judith Hunter. 2006. "Family Centred Care: A Review of Qualitative Studies." *Journal of Clinical Nursing* 15(10): 1317–23.

Annie's Problem

JACKIE LEACH SCULLY

Annie has a problem. Her brother Stewart has been on dialysis for kidney disease for many years, and his condition has started to deteriorate. When the option of a related member of the family giving him a healthy kidney came up, two of his three siblings were ready and willing to donate (although his younger brother, Martin, was a little more reluctant). To their disappointment, however, neither Annie nor her sister Louise turned out to be a suitable match for Stewart.

It was then they were told there was a way around this: they could enter a pool of possible donor matches. If the computer found suitable crossmatches to either Annie or Louise, they could donate a kidney to an unknown recipient on the list, while someone else from the pool donated a suitable kidney to Stewart. The end result, the transplant nurse smilingly assures Annie, is exactly the same: she donates a kidney, and Stewart receives. It's just that they don't do it to each other.

It looks the same, it sounds the same. But to Annie, it doesn't feel the same. She tries to explain her feelings to the nurse, who seems to misunderstand her worries and starts once again to go through the risks of the procedure with her. To Annie, it isn't the risks that are the problem here, but she isn't quite clear what is. She leaves the conversation with the nurse feeling uneasy and continues to worry about it over the next few weeks. She wants to help Stewart, and she doesn't want him or the rest of the family to think that she's reluctant to take whatever measures are necessary to do so. But this kind of donation just isn't the same. Is it?

Annie is confronted here with several problems, interacting with each other. Indirectly, through Stewart's illness, she faces the societal problem that there is a large and growing gap between the number of people in need of organ transplantation (kidney being the most common) and the number of organs available from cadavers. As a result, transplant services in several countries have been introducing novel routes through which organs can be donated by living persons. Live donation has the added advantage that it tends to give better results, with fewer immunological problems, than cadaveric transplantation. There are now essentially three types of living organ donation: (1) directed donation to a known relative (genetic or what is often described as "emotional" donation), which is what Annie had in mind for her donation to Stewart; (2) altruistic donation by a healthy person to a stranger, who fortuitously is a suitable match—which, it seems from the scenario we've outlined, is not an option for Stewart; and (3) nondirected, paired, or pooled donation schemes. It's one of these that is being suggested to Annie.

Paired donation schemes have been established relatively recently in a number of countries, including the US and Korea, and in the UK since the introduction of the Human Tissue Act 2006 (Johnson et al. 2006). Here, Annie and Stewart are paired with another donor–recipient couple (let's say John and Alex, who are perhaps partners, parent and child, or siblings) who are also willing enough to donate and receive, but are incompatible. The crucial point would be that donor John is compatible with recipient Stewart, and Annie with Alex. So Annie gives her kidney to Alex, and Stewart gets his from John.

Pooled donation makes things significantly more complicated. These schemes encompass a variety of different structures, but essentially the incompatible donor–recipient pairs enter a "pool" of potential matches. Say that while Annie is compatible with Alex, unfortunately it turns out that John can't donate to Stewart—but he can to someone else in the pool, Hilary, and it so happens that Hilary's willing-but-incompatible donor, Hester, is compatible with Stewart. Once possible combinations of matches have been identified and all pairs are in agreement, Annie's kidney goes to Alex, John's to Hilary, and Hester's to Stewart. Pooled donation can include pairs and single altruistic donors, in a chain of interventions where in principle the only limits to the number of links are the practicalities of identifying the potential pairs and of setting up a number of simultaneous transplant operations. In the UK since the Human Tissue Act came into force, both two-way paired and three-way pooled transplants have taken place. On the face of it, the schemes are promising solutions (or at least partial solutions) to the sociomedical problem of donor scarcity.

The ethical issues raised by cadaver organ donation and, increasingly, by living related or unrelated donation have been well rehearsed (see, among many others, Miller and Truog 2011). Some distinctive problems have been recognized as associated with living donation. For the physician, the removal of a kidney from a healthy donor runs counter to the professional principle of not exposing a patient to avoidable risk ("First, do no harm"): in donor nephrectomy, a surgeon exposes a healthy person to risk to save the life of someone else. Present-day procedures mean that the risk of death to the donor is low (0.03%), and so is the risk of life-threatening or disabling complications such as pulmonary embolism or myocardial infarction (0.23%). What are generally referred to as less serious complications are more common, running at around 8 percent, although it may be questioned to what extent pneumonia or wound infection should be classed as "less serious."

A primary ethical concern about living donation to a known person has always been the potential for coercion, however implicit or benign. It's precisely the strength of the ties between biologically or emotionally related family members that can make it impossible to refuse a loved one's request for a kidney, even when there are legitimate reasons for caution. Potential donors may have particular anxieties about the operation or its consequences, either for themselves or their own dependents. It's important to recognize that, although invasive surgery is increasingly normalized in our society, these anxieties are not irrational: surgery can be painful, anesthesia is not without risk, long-term complications do sometimes happen, and whether they do or not, the disruption to the donor's own life plans can be significant.

Feminist bioethicists have also drawn attention to the pattern of gender imbalance that has been observed within living organ donation. Donation of organs from women to men seems to happen significantly more often than from men to women, or male–male/female–female donations (see, e.g., Steinman 2006; Thompson et al. 2003). The data are not always clear, and there can also be reasonable clinical grounds for why men are more likely to be recipients in living donation. Nevertheless, there remains a residual concern that what may be operating here are assumptions about the compassionate, "giving" role of women, and their traditional responsibility to care for the health of the family breadwinner.

Annie may face one or both of these recognized ethical problems. It doesn't sound from our scenario as if either Annie or her sister Louise are facing any overt coercion. On the other hand, it may be impossible to accurately spot the point at which reasonable anticipation of Annie's willingness, based on this family's history of relationship and exchanges, slides into a weight of expectation that is effectively a form of benign coercion. It does seem that one sibling, Martin, has been able to express his reservations without apparently damaging his relationships with the rest of the family. The fact that the two sisters are the ones who have been willing to go further along the road to donation may trigger some concerns about imbalanced gendered expectations here.

But the problem that Annie has tried, and so far failed, to articulate is of a different ethical order from these. Primarily—and this is one of the central arguments of this collection—it seems to arise from the discordance between the sorts of ethical relationships and perspectives that exist within a family and those that govern the behavior of the healthcare system dealing with those families. For living related and unrelated donation where problems of blood group or histoincompatibility are common, the move to achieving the same goal (two or more people in need receive a healthy kidney) but indirectly (via donors who happen to be more compatible) is a logical one. Moreover, it is structurally the same. Whether done directly or indirectly, Annie gives a kidney and Stewart receives one. (Indeed, looking beyond Annie's own family, it is arguably better than direct donation, since the end result is two people receiving kidneys who otherwise would not.)

From the viewpoint of the transplant scheme, the significant step was Annie's first consent, to donate a kidney to Stewart. Entry into a paired or pooled scheme is an alternative way of achieving this, so Annie's "yes" to the original question of donation still holds. Of course, the clinical team would not formally take this for granted and would be expected to seek Annie's informed consent to entering into the pooled scheme. But it can seem counterintuitive to them that she might feel ready to say "yes" to one pathway to donation but less able to do so to the other. Here's Annie, talking to her best friend Jack:

It wasn't even until we were five or ten minutes into the chat that I realized the nurse was talking about something really different, and I asked her to go back through it all over again. She was talking about how long it might take to find a match in the pool and she just seemed to take it for granted that I'd be okay about that. So I said I wanted some time to think about it, and she asked me what the problem was. When I said, "Well, it's very different from just giving Stew my kidney," she seemed a bit taken aback. She kept saying no, the risks and everything are the same. She gave me some leaflets and let me go away to think about it but I could tell she wasn't happy.

From Annie's point of view, there are some important factors that contribute to the feeling that giving a kidney to her brother is so obviously what she should do and wants to do, and for her, these factors are significantly different in a paired or pooled scheme from what they are in direct donation. Of course she still wants to help her brother, but this way of doing it is not the same in an embodied or an emotional sense. An important thing about donation to Stewart is the embodied connection: her kidney, her own tissue, a part of herself, takes up residence in and becomes part of her brother.

But even more fundamentally than that, what makes donation of her kidney even thinkable in the first place is that it is to someone in emotional and/or biological relationship to her. Annie would never have contemplated being an altruistic donor to an unknown stranger. Donation to a relative or partner, on the other hand is, well, just something that you do, because you know them and you love them. People might have very understandable fears about the pain of the surgery, or complications from it, but the current social expectation would still come down on the side of donation as the norm in these circumstances. In most families (or, at least, as we would like to imagine most families being), the instinctive response to a brother in need of a kidney transplant would be to offer to be a donor. Of course this expectation is not uniform: other relevant factors that would change the weight of expectation would be the potential donor's own health, responsibilities they might have to others in the family. Martin, for instance, could be reluctant to be considered a donor in the first place because he feels his overriding responsibility is to his own children: What if he dies as a result of the operation, or what if one of them needs a kidney from him at some point in the future? Nor is it clear where the contours of expectation fade away completely, and whether these map onto genetic, emotional, or some other index of relatedness.

Nevertheless, Annie is left trying to account for and justify her intuition to herself, the transplant team, and perhaps even Stewart. Here she is again, over a glass of wine with Jack:

> It was obvious to me right from the start that if I was a match for Stew, he'd have my kidney. That's a complete no-brainer. I did think about the risks, but they'd have to be a lot worse to come anywhere near making me think again. But this is one step removed. It feels like giving my kidney to a stranger, and I admire people who do that, but it's not something I'd ever think of doing. I do understand it's all the same in the end if Stew gets a kidney, but this is kind of halfway between a stranger and my brother, and it feels like I'm being pushed towards something I'd never wanted to do. And, anyway, because it's "you give me yours, I'll give you mine," it feels a bit like a trade, and I'm really uncomfortable with that. How long is it before they say, "Oh, well, the pool hasn't worked, but how about we sell you one for 2,000 quid?"

REFERENCES

Johnson, Rachel J., Joanne E. Allen, Susan V. Fuggle, Andrew J. Bradley, and Chris Rudge, on behalf of the Kidney Advisory Group, UK Transplant (NHSBT). 2008. "Early Experience of Paired Living Kidney Donation in the United Kingdom." *Transplantation* 86: 1672–77.

Miller, Franklin G., and Robert Truog. 2011. *Death, Dying and Organ Transplantation.* Oxford: Oxford University Press.

Steinman, Judith L. 2006. "Gender Disparity in Organ Donation." *Gender Medicine* 3: 246–52.

Thompson, Teresa L., James D. Robinson, and R. Wade Kenny. 2003. "Gender Differences in Family Communication About Organ Donation." *Sex Roles* 49: 587–96.

Chapter 5

Justice, Intimacy, and Autonomy

JAMIE LINDEMANN NELSON AND SIMON WOODS

Rawls tells us that "justice is the first virtue of social institutions, as truth is of systems of thought" (1971, 3), and it might be thought that if ever anyone was, he is surely entitled to an opinion. If he's right, though, families are even odder instances of social institutions than they may otherwise appear; indeed, perhaps the small scale of family life, coupled with the character of the relations and reasons often found within it, keep families from being proper social institutions at all, at least as Rawls employs the notion. Familial intimacy and love are distinguishable from—and may be flatly incompatible with—the kind of relationships and motivations that justice is often taken to presuppose; the freedom families have to transfer resources, training, and traditions from generation to generation may frustrate justice's ambitions to keep inequality in check.

The problems we grapple with in this chapter are set by these ways in which families vex contemporary understandings of justice—as well as how those understandings pose problems for families. We aim both to provide an overview of the tensions among various specifications of justice and practices characteristic of families and to explore in greater detail two sites where those tensions erupt into conspicuous problems. The overall goal is to get a firmer grasp on how justice bears on both relationships within families and relationships between families and what is clearly a significant social institution, healthcare.

Justice as a general concept is characterized variously, but it seems fair to say that a notion close to its core is that treating people differently, at least with respect to parts of their lives that are not trivial, requires some relevant distinction among them that shows why the different treatment is not morally arbitrary. Current discussions parse justice in a number of ways. *Distributive justice*, for example, concerns what (if any) differences among people—differences in effort, for example, or in need, or in productivity—justify different apportionments of such benefits as income and wealth (Rawls 1971). *Contributive justice* addresses the reasons for which chances to engage in and enrich social life may be made available or withheld (Calder n.d.; Gomberg 2007). *Epistemic justice* assesses how people are afforded or denied opportunities to be heard and credited in public and private discourse (Fricker 2009; Dotson 2014). *Recognitional justice* inspects how various ways in which people mark their identities—for example, via ethnicity, gender, class, sexual preference, the generation into which they were born, or how their bodies function—are socially acknowledged, ignored, or repudiated (Frazer 1997). Further, the complex and interwoven ways in which some groups of people have been characteristically treated unjustly are treated by some theorists as distinctive categories (say, gender justice, racial justice).

Other specifications of justice (e.g., retributive, transitional, restorative, transformational) are observed as well, although more commonly in connection with criminal than with social justice. They tend, therefore, to presuppose, rather than to interrogate or motivate, ongoing accounts of what sort of differences among people or groups are salient morally. However, *restorative* justice and possibly its sibling, *transformative* justice, appear to have both aspirations and methods that are specifically relevant to many forms of family. Both are characterized by their concern with responding to acts of injustice as instances of damage to the community as well as to individuals within it, but *not*—or, at least, not primarily—to the state, whose responses to such acts are generally seen as disproportionate and biased, carceral, and otherwise violent, and all too frequently, ineffectual when not counterproductive. Community response fostered by restorative justice aims at healing injury, acknowledging harms, taking responsibility (including community as well as perpetrator responsibility) for their infliction, and allowing diverse forms of compensation, all in the service of determining how the affected parties—victims, perpetrators, citizens in general—can find the terms with which to go on together after the damage that has been done (Braithwaite 2002).

As the community in question might be a family, this approach might seem well suited to responding to injustices that may occur within them. Consider, for instance, a family in which one of the children has been abused by a sibling. The family aims to respond in a way that does justice to all concerned: to acknowledge and mourn and try to heal or at least to mitigate the trauma undergone by the victim and the lesser but real harms suffered by the family and its members: the shattering of trust, the imperiling of affection. It also needs to act to restore safety and security in the family both as sensibility and due to better practices of guard and support, ideally in ways that may allow everyone in the family the opportunity to go on with one another as family, in some sense of that term.

Yet both restorative theory and practice need development here—the literature in this area repeatedly warns about the special dangers that come with using restorative techniques within families facing issues of domestic abuse (Zehr 2014). Including families within the ambit of justice adds complications not just to restorative approaches, but throughout this array. Consider (as we will do in some detail later in the chapter) those families who are caring intensively for relatives with profound healthcare needs: getting straight about their claims to social support requires determining whether duties of care within families might lessen or cancel those claims—while at the same time staying alert to the social value of family-based care, and of families themselves.

Consider the stress placed on some healthcare systems by those subfertile people who turn to medicine hoping to start or extend families. Given existing children seeking parental care—indeed, given the environmental impact of each person born into high-consumptive economies (Conley 2016)—pronatalist attitudes and practices are in urgent need of compelling justification. In particular, the question "what is there about having a biological connection between parents and children that warrants using public health care resources for the purpose?" wants a better answer than those currently in play.

Questions about social support for family-provided healthcare or for assisted reproduction, however motivated, clearly involve distributive justice. Yet these and other questions that arise when families are caught up in professional healthcare involve other subgenres of justice too—the example in the previous paragraph suggests that issues of environmental justice can be pertinent. Consider also disputes about the appropriate role of parents in authorizing their children's participation in medical research, construed as a matter of permissibility, and the range of parental authority in the classic Ramsey–McCormick debates of the mid-1970s (Ramsey 1976; McCormick 1976) may be seen through a different normative lens when contributive justice is taken into account. Children may sometimes have a right to participate, and parents in some circumstances have a duty to facilitate their doing so. Should people with disabilities be involved in women's decisions about whether to continue pregnancies where prenatal testing reveals fetal anomalies, or with parental decisions concerning newborns or children with impairments? Here, recognitional justice is pitted against the prerogative sometimes asserted by parents or other adult members to determine central features of how a family conducts itself, sometimes referred to as "parental" or "family" autonomy (Fishkin 1983). Do family care providers' accounts of their ill or incapacitated relatives—maybe distorted by affection and ignorance of healthcare, maybe sharpened by affection and understanding of the patient—get appropriate uptake and acknowledgment from professional providers, or is the epistemic standpoint of these family members belittled, subjecting them to "testimonial injustice" (Fricker 2009)?

In all of these cases, the importance of appeals to justice is complicated by the patterns of intimacy that characterize many families. While we don't expect to resolve any of those complications here, we do aim to contribute to a better appreciation of their intricacy by exploring a feature of many discussions of justice and a widely held view about the particular moral standing of families.

This is the view referred to above as "family autonomy." It holds that the integrity and value of families requires some degree of insulation from the authority of some general moral norms, including justice; the way families are allowed to impart skills and other resources between generations, mentioned earlier in the chapter, is often used as a primary example, as it preserves class inequities that many understandings of distributive justice find distinctly troublesome.

While family autonomy gestures in the direction of an important feature of the relation between families and general moral norms, we are dissatisfied with how it portrays that relationship. "Family autonomy" may convey an image of families seen as individual moral agents, modeled after notions of the self distorted by an exaggerated conception of individualism. Indeed, the idea that a family's activities are to some degree exempt from standing moral norms that govern human interactions generally displays a particularly extreme version of that atomistic view; autonomy as a morally significant property of individuals is often touted as the *basis* for people's being both protected by and beholden to moral norms. In any event, we here proceed on an understanding of familial prerogatives to order their own affairs that doesn't claim that they are excused from the full rigor of certain moral norms. Rather, we see family prerogatives as resting in part on the point that what it is for a given family to flourish, in all its particularity of personalities, histories, and traditions, may require some variance from normative conceptions operative on largely more impersonal scales. While we don't suggest that sincerity alone justifies whatever practices authoritative members of families put in place, within a broad understanding of reasonableness, we think that a family's own conception of its good has a claim to forbearance, even should it conflict with such wider norms. "Reasonableness" will turn out to be highly sensitive to particular features of families and the social contexts in which they are situated, but ought as a general matter to include acknowledgment of dissent and diverging interests within families, including appropriate exit options.

None of this is to deny that tensions can arise between some of the ways in which justice is understood with respect to the overall structure of social life, and how justice and other moral norms are conceived within families. Our discussion of these tensions will be illustrated by parental refusal of appropriate vaccinations for their children. First, though, we address the claim that justice is relevant only in certain material and motivational circumstances, by examining how specific features of families complicate questions of distributive justice in the support of intensive family-based care provision.

I. THE "CIRCUMSTANCES OF JUSTICE," FAMILIAL INTIMACY, AND FAMILY MEMBERS AS HEALTHCARE PROVIDERS

Since Hume, many have thought that justice is relevant to guide action only if certain background conditions obtain (Hope 2010). This notion—the "circumstances of justice"—seems particularly pertinent to justice in distribution. Egalitarians, for example, tend to think any departure from equality in each person's holdings or welfare requires extensive justification; libertarians, by contrast, will ask how a given distribution came about and in principle will accept any arrangement, so long as it arose from transfers free of force or fraud from initial holdings justly acquired (Nozick 1974).

These and other conceptions require that conditions of "moderate scarcity" prevail if justice is to make much moral sense. Under conditions of absolute scarcity, there would be nothing to distribute, while in conditions of superabundance, there seems no need to deliberate about just distribution at all; there would be more than enough to satisfy everyone.

It is fair to point out that other norms presuppose certain circumstances, too: honesty, for example, requires both that we *can* communicate our thoughts to one another and that we are *not* transparent to each other. Otherwise, insisting on honesty would seem rather beside the point. The virtue of hope requires the ability to envisage the future; the imperative of reparation, the ability to remember the past. And so on.

Yet justice's ties to circumstances seem to involve less generic features of life. Apart from needing certain material states of affairs—which are, admittedly, likely to obtain—the required psychological abilities are far from guaranteed, and may not always be appropriate. Whether or not ethics as such requires impartiality, for instance, the ability to deliberate without playing favorites seems internally connected to justice. Yet people do not typically regard the interests of their family members as though they were simply one collection of morally considerable beings among many others. Further, leading conceptions of justice—and surely of distributive justice—tend to portray people as mutually disinterested. However accurate this presupposition may be among strangers, it hardly seems suited to intimates.

Parents, for example, incline to see the interests of their children not simply as external constraints to be avoided if possible and accommodated if necessary, but as among their own interests too— direct reasons for their actions, as well as for their children's actions. Behavior that seems self-sacrificial from the point of view of mutually disinterested strangers, and therefore from that of justice, may well seem perfectly natural or even necessary among close relatives.

How families fit within justice's circumstances, then, is unclear. Few families enjoy superabundance and many escape absolute scarcity; hence, the material considerations are satisfied. Yet when it comes to motivational considerations, matters are more problematic. On the one hand, even close-knit, well-functioning families—indeed, perhaps *especially* such families—have concerns about fairness and exploitation in how responsibilities are assigned; on the other, family members don't typically stand on their rights when their relatives face pressing needs. Neither do they customarily coordinate family life by hammering out deals that assume that each party is indifferent to the interests of the others.

And yet concerns about unfairness, exploitation, and what would ordinarily be called injustice in families abide. A conspicuous example: women continue to take on the brunt of domestic responsibilities, even when they work at full-time jobs outside the home (Hochschild and Machung 2012). When difficult healthcare responsibilities fall on families, similar patterns persist; while men do more than in past years, US-based studies find that between 59%

and 75% of those providing care to relatives with health deficits are female (Kaiser Family Fund 2002; Doty 2010; National Alliance for Caregiving and AARP 2009).

How, then, are we to conceptualize the apparent injustice that goes on within families, given how awkwardly they fit with the circumstances of justice? This is an important question, not merely for families seeking to get their own affairs in better order but also for health and social policy, which have allowed families to take on increasingly challenging caregiving responsibilities in recent years. In the US, for example, over 40 million Americans are estimated to be caring for a relative who needs help with at least one "activity of daily living" in their homes; the economic value of family-provided healthcare was estimated to be over $450 billion in 2009 (Feinberg et al., 2011). A study in the UK found that the value of the work of unpaid caregivers exceeded that of the entire NHS budget (Buckner et al. 2011). The role of such labor within healthcare systems hardly goes unnoticed and is subject to debate, perhaps particularly in Europe, Yet even so, the level of scrutiny and controversy it prompts seems mismatched to what would otherwise count as a massive impressment of unpaid workers into difficult and sometimes nasty and damaging work.

Why? A reasonable hypothesis is the widespread conviction that providing care is just the sort of thing that people in families are there to do for each other—a conviction that many caregiving family members, and not only health policy makers, seem to share. Family members are often willing, and sometimes eager, to provide healthcare for their families, even if other possibilities for responding to a relative's need are available (although attitudes seem sensitive to, *inter alia,* the age and gender of the care provider, and to the character of the illness (Reinhardt et al, 2008)). Some family members may experience care provision as what Harry Frankfurt has called a "volitional necessity"—which is to say that the opportunity to care is experienced not as a choice, subject to the balance of costs and benefits, but as a course of action to which a person simply must commit herself because doing so is a condition of the coherence of her sense of self (Frankfurt 1989).

Volitional necessities would appear to be rife in families. It might seem to follow that there's no offense against justice *within* a family, however we are to understand that idea, if someone is suffered to do as she feels she must. Does it further follow that the state may justly allow people to care for their ill relatives boundlessly, adjusting health funding and insurance schemes to take full advantage of this motivation, no matter how many homes come to resemble hospital wards, nor how many wives and husbands, sons and daughters, sisters and brothers become nurses and health technicians *manqué*?

There are reasons to think that it does not. Despite the importance of caregiving provided by "husbands, sons, and brothers," the persisting gender imbalances in the provision of care suggest that something other than familial love pure and simple is at work. The gap suggests that some of the values and desires that go into a family member's self-conception as a primary caregiver are adaptive rather than authentic—psychic accommodations to bad (unjust) circumstances, rather than expressions of personality unfettered by indefensible constraints (Khader 2011). Grant that many people cannot coherently conceive of themselves as parents apart from intensely loving their children, and that such love is internally connected with an intense desire to care for them. It remains reasonable to ask why the way that love plays out in many families should place sterner burdens on female than on male parents, and to note the correlations between those burdens and the multiple ways in which women's participation in social life is constricted and undervalued.

Accepting that distribution of responsibilities within families may be unjust, despite their intimacy and penchant for partiality, may prompt a better characterization of what justice is, as well as of the circumstances that are its proper background. So doing may also open up space for families to have justice-based claims against the state for caregiving support that explicitly accommodate their own caregiving responsibilities. From the perspective of family members themselves, however, a decent case for social support of their health-care provision may not need to wait on a more sophisticated understanding of how justice and intimacy relate. Even family members who authentically feel that their very identities are implicated in the exacting care they provide for their ill parents or children, spouses or siblings, may be glad of help. Regular and reliable respite care, ready opportunities for consultation with professionals, and subvention for caregiving costs, including lost income, need not threaten anyone's integrity or hamper their flourishing. Given the persistence of conspicuous gender imbalances in the distribution of caring labor in families, such support serves ends valued by societies that aspire to be just.

Yet to show that social support is compatible with respecting what families may experience as imperatives to care and contribute to the ends of social justice leaves open how much support justice demands. It's helpful, then, to understand the magnitude of the harms families can incur in prolonged, intensive, and ill-supported caring work (e.g., Grunfield et al. 2004; Chen, 2014). As a recent European study found:

> The availability of and burden on family carers are increasingly pressing concerns for public health given the rising old-age dependency ratio, increasing geographic mobility, changes in traditional family structures, urbanization and the growing participation of women in the labour market. The trend towards end-of-life care in the community may also put additional financial strain on patients at the end of life and on their families, as

it is likely to cause a shift in cost burden away from public health care systems and towards patients and families. Research indicates that family carers of dying people experience a wide range of unmet needs, physical and emotional strains and financial burden. (Pivodic et al. 2014)

Such intense healthcare provision can seriously hamper a caregiver's chances to contribute to and benefit from social life, violating a state's commitment to equality of opportunity—a relatively weak conception of equality to which even the US is officially bound. For example, family care providers can lose the chance to compete fairly for desirable positions for which they have inclination and talent but lack the time and energy needed for gaining training or experience. What is more, their chances for other forms of self-maintenance and self-development can be diminished or lost as well; if the "opportunity" the equal opportunity principle addresses includes chances to grow as an emotional and reflective being, as well as an economic one, this is a significant loss.

Illness doesn't imperil only some individual conception of a good life, but virtually all of them. Health, therefore, doesn't serve merely some individuals' conception of what is good—it serves almost every reasonable conception of what is worth pursuing in life, and is thus what Norman Daniels, following Rawls, has called a "primary good" (Daniels 1985). But the impact of providing long periods of exacting healthcare to family members might be analogized to the impact of being ill itself. The data suggest that prolonged provision of exacting care seems intriguingly analogous to illness in just these wide-scale ways: the taxes of time, energy, and health that it can levy threaten a range of human goods that seem almost equally numerous and rich.

Further, if the burdens facing family caregivers have not been appropriately reckoned, the benefits they provide may be misunderstood as well. To the extent that public health and caring for the ill are seen as generating social and not merely private goods, there is further reason to take care that the costs of discharging the responsibilities and obtaining those goods are equitably distributed (Olsaretti 2013). It also needs to be borne in mind that the intensity of the challenges involved in family care provision is not solely a fact of nature. It stems in part from many social decisions, including agendas for medical research. Surely, most welcome the overall impact of that research on mortality. But it has had its "externalities" as well: resultant extended care needs that fall not only on patients but often on their families as well.

It is on the basis of considerations of this sort, then, that we hold that family caregiving has a valid, justice-based claim to social support. This hardly qualifies as a radical conclusion: in many countries, even including the US, *some* provisions for caregivers are made. The live questions concern how burdensome caregiving needs to be to justify what kinds of state support. Might opening questions of this sort suggest that some families may not be doing their "fair share," and not only deserve no state-supplied resources but should be encouraged or directed to care further, drawing on their internal resources until some threshold is reached? What might be said of the deserts of two families, both caring for a seriously and chronically ill loved one, but faring very differently as caregivers and as families because of differences in their organizational abilities or their inherent psychological resilience? Are the comparative deficits of the family that finds itself continually over its head grounds for providing them with more support than the family that copes well? Does society have a right to expect a certain baseline level of competence in family caregiving abilities, or does such a question (along with concepts such as "inherent psychological resilience") wrongly obscure the social conditions that promote or undermine such abilities and dispositions?

II. "FAMILY AUTONOMY" AND PROXY
DECISION MAKING: VACCINE REFUSAL

Questions about what challenges to families ought to trigger what kind of resources will need to take caregiver burdens on families, their equitable distribution within families, and the social sources of and social benefits of that caring with greater seriousness. The question of public scrutiny of family caregiving practices will also need to reckon with the question of "family autonomy." If part of the argument for social support of family caregiving is that the benefits it accords are not altogether private, it could seem that society has further reason to vet the quality of the care that goes on in families. The default assumption prevailing widely—at least as respects families who are otherwise privileged within their social order—that family caregiving is provided consistently enough and competently enough so that no regular formal assessment is required is another expression of the norm that families (the "good ones," in any event) are to enjoy considerable leeway in ordering themselves.

Familial caregiving practices do sometimes come under closer public scrutiny in healthcare settings. Professional providers have both legal and moral responsibilities to safeguard the well-being of their patients, in ways that may conflict with how caregivers and decision makers understand the proper distribution of burdens and benefits within their families. In much of the world, family proxy decision makers are instructed not to take account of anyone's interests apart from the patient's; any effect treatment decisions may have on family members is irrelevant (Hardart and Truog 2003). Decisions emerging from families to withdraw or withhold treatment from newborn members, for example, might well trigger contestation and legal challenge by professional providers, either because the professionals think that the family's deliberations have not been focused solely on the patient or because the family disagrees with decisions made solely with the patient's good in view.

However, when the stakes are not quite so stark as they might be in the NICU, there are areas in which the prerogative of parents to make healthcare decisions for their children remains extensive. Consider the anti-vaccination movement.

In the US, children must undergo a battery of injections to start or stay in public school, absent either medical *or* "philosophical" exceptions. Some skepticism about vaccines has persisted since their introduction, but it had been fairly muted in recent years (Stern and Markel 2005). The upsurge of resistance in the US, the UK, and elsewhere is in no small part attributable to an article published in *The Lancet* in 1998 by the British physician Alex Wakefield and colleagues, noting correlations between MMR vaccine administration and the incidence of autism. That article has since been much assailed and was withdrawn by *The Lancet* in 2010. However, the incidence of vaccination in the US and the UK has since dropped to levels that in some areas threaten the robustness of herd immunity.

Parents who press for philosophical exemptions from vaccine requirements are usually not chiefly motivated by the bare desire to assert their autonomy from social norms, nor even solely by conformity to norms resident in the communities with which they most strongly identify. Often they are moved by concern about their children's health. If the issue were to be conceived of strictly in terms of family autonomy, it would be appropriate to ask how absolute a conception of the notion ought to be in play, either in general or with respect to the specific issue. Thinking of a family's prerogatives in terms of reasonable conceptions of its flourishing, however, may shift attention from a general, rather abstract level closer to the consideration of what might be said in favor of a family's reasons for its position.

In vaccine cases, there may be reasons worth hearing. While the allegations of a causal link between vaccines and autism are almost surely false, vaccination is not altogether without some very small risk of serious, even mortal harm. If a family lives in an area where the anti-vaccine movement is not strong, the parents can rely on robust herd immunity to protect their children from measles, mumps, rubella, whooping cough, and so forth, without subjecting them to the risk posed by vaccines. If parents decide on this basis, therefore, to try for a philosophical exemption (or can send their kids to a private school), should their decision be respected as proceeding from deliberations reflecting a family's reasonable notion of what best promotes its own flourishing?

It might be argued that families typically expose their children on a routine basis to many tiny threats of deadly harm—swimming lessons, contact sports, putting them on the school bus. Why balk at inoculation? At the same time, the fact that parents are allowed to expose their kids to such risks routinely might be cited in support of seeing vaccine refusal as a protected expression of a family's prerogative to order its affairs according to a reasonable conception of its good. One can't learn to swim without going into the water, but one can be safe from infectious disease absent the risk of vaccination (at least, as long as families are willing to be thoughtful about their travel plans).

Granted their premises, the strongest reply to such a family would seem to be an appeal to justice. They are proposing to "free ride" on the risks and discomforts other families accept, to protect their kids by the sacrifices made by others without participating themselves in that sacrifice. Given the actual situation confronting our imagined families— robust herd immunity, the remote possibility that a child could die as a result of an intervention that in any event will be unpleasant and may not help them at all—why doesn't the allowable degree of parental partiality for their own children justify the continuance of philosophical exemptions?

The free rider objection to this hypothetical family's proposal looks rather like a confrontation between family autonomy and justice *sans phrase*. The parents wish to have their children treated differently from others, but with no clearly relevant moral distinction between them. Yet forcing compliance could be damaging to a family's own structures of authority, to say nothing of traumatizing children for reasons that are likely to benefit them not at all.

Perhaps the conflict can be finessed away. It's often thought that the best response to parents who resist having their children vaccinated is education. Explain the risks and benefits in a clear way, and *voilà*, rational persuasion is achieved and the kids will get their vaccinations without any need to determine whether free riding justifies overriding a family's prerogative to determine its own schedule of risks and benefits.

The difficulty with this plan is that experience suggests it doesn't work. In fact, expanding on the risks of childhood illnesses has a tendency to be counterproductive. While questions exist concerning the quality of the research that gives rise to what is taught, as well as regarding the quality of the teaching itself, recent work suggests that a reluctant family's hesitations are often entrenched and cannot be removed by instructional efforts (Nyhan et al., 2014).

What does seem to work is, in effect, to take the decision out of the family's hands by treating vaccination simply as a matter of routine. Parents are informed, but not asked for their consent. If they want to prevent their children from being vaccinated, they can, but there is no explicit opportunity provided them to do so (McCarthy 2015).

On its face, this strategy looks set to collide with epistemic justice. It assumes that parents are either fully on board with the perspective of care providers, and therefore it is superfluous to require explicit consent for vaccination, or they are not, in which case it would be wrong to ask them to consent. Such parents are not regarded as epistemically respectworthy—they can't be trusted to handle information properly, and are emphatically not seen as people whose judgments regarding their children's health should be taken into account, at least not in this respect.

This seems a typical justification when powerful institutions seek to condition people's access to information: those denied are alleged to be incapable of handling it responsibly. The question this strategy leaves us with is whether and when a policy that explicitly embraces manipulating people can be a way of increasing healthcare compliance that is consistent with treating people justly as knowers. Perhaps the manipulation of parents is a more defensible version of this practice, as the well-being of whole communities, as well as children, is at risk. Yet perhaps it is less so, as it not only attacks an individual's self-regarding interests but also preempts parents' responsibilities and prerogatives with respect to their children, on the grounds that "doctor knows best."

III. CONCLUSION

Justice, as Hume saw it, is a "cautious, jealous virtue." Most, however, like to think of families as homes for virtues less cramped, for whatever abilities we have to be moved by the interests of others to flourish. In real worlds, of course, there is plenty of jealousy, and even some reason for caution, in families, which is why, along with more expansive norms of care and affection, justice is needed within them, as well as between them and other institutions. Yet to get a better purchase on the distributive and epistemic questions touched on here, as well as matters of recognition, contribution, and many others left unexplored, social theorizing needs to pay attention to a wider range of human interaction than may have been done by Hume or by Rawls. If families need to accommodate the demands of justice, justice may have to return the favor.

ACKNOWLEDGMENT

We thank Gideon Calder for his extensive, searching, and generous comments on a late draft.

REFERENCES

Braithwaite, John. 2002. *Restorative Justice and Responsive Regulation.* Oxford: Oxford University Press.

Buckner, Lisa, Sue Yeandle, and Carers UK. 2011. "Valuing Carers: Calculating the Value of Carers' Support." http://www.carersuk.org/media/k2/attachments/Valuing_carers_2011___Carers_UK.pdf

Calder, Gideon. n.d. "The Family, Inter-Generational Inequality, and Contributive Injustice."

Chen, Mei-Lan. 2016. "The Growing Costs and Burden of Family Caregiving of Older Adults: A Review of Paid Sick Leave and Family Leave Policies." *The Gerontologist* 56(3): 391–96.

Conley, Sarah. 2016. *One Child.* Oxford and New York: Oxford University Press.

Daniels, Norman. 1985. *Just Health Care.* Cambridge, UK, and New York: Cambridge University Press.

Dotson, Kristie. 2014. "Conceptualizing Epistemic Oppression." *Social Epistemology* 28(2): 115–38.

Doty, Pamela. 2010. "The Evolving Balance of Formal and Informal, Institutional and Non-Institutional Long-Term Care for Older Americans: A Thirty-Year Perspective." *Public Policy & Aging Report* 20(1): 3–9.

Feinberg, Lynn, Susan C. Reinhard, Ari Houser, and Rita Choula. 2011. *Valuing the Invaluable.* AARP Public Policy Institute. http://assets.aarp.org/rgcenter/ppi/ltc/i51-caregiving.pdf, accessed March 27, 2015.

Fishkin, James S. 1983. *Justice, Equal Opportunity, and the Family*. New Haven, CT: Yale University Press.

Frankfurt, Harry G. 1989. *The Importance of What We Care About*. New York and Cambridge, UK: Cambridge University Press,

Fraser, Nancy. 1997. "From Redistribution to Recognition." In *Justice Interruptus*. London and New York: Routledge.

Fricker, Miranda. 2009. *Epistemic Injustice*. Oxford and New York: Oxford University Press.

Gomberg, Paul. 2007. *How to Make Opportunity Equal: Race and Contributive Justice*. Oxford: Blackwell.

Grunfield, E., D. Coyle, T. Whelan, J. Clinch, L. Reyno, C. C. Earle, A. Willan, R. Viola, M. Coristine, T. Janz, and R. Glossop. 2004 "Family Caregiver Burden: Results of a Longitudinal Study of Breast Cancer Patients and Their Principal Caregivers." *Canadian Medical Association Journal* 170(12): 1795–801.

Hardart, George E., and Robert D. Truog. 2003. "Attitudes and Preferences of Intensivists Regarding the Role of Family Interests in Medical Decision Making for Incompetent Patients." *Critical Care Medicine* 31(7): 1895–990.

Hochschild, Arlie, and Anne Machung. 2012. *The Second Shift*. New York: Penguin.

Henry J. Kaiser Family Foundation (KFF), Harvard School of Public Health, United Hospital Fund of New York, and Visiting Nurse Service of New York. 2002. *The Wide Circle of Caregiving: Key Findings from a National Survey: Long-Term Care from the Caregiver's Perspective*. Menlo Park, NJ: KFF.

Hope, Simon. "The Circumstances of Justice." *Hume Studies* 36(2): 125–8.

Khader, Serenej. 2011. *Adaptive Preferences and Women's Empowerment*. Oxford and New York: Oxford University Press.

McCarthy, C. 2015. "A Sticky Decision: Should Parents Be Obligated to Vaccinate?" Lecture presented at the "Families Matter" conference, Harvard Medical School, March 19, 2015.

McCormick, Richard A. 1976. "Experimentation in Children: Sharing in Sociality." *Hastings Center Report* 6(6): 41–46.

National Alliance for Caregiving and AARP. 2009. *Caregiving in the U.S.* Washington, DC: National Alliance for Caregiving.

Nozick, Robert. 1974. *Anarchy, State, and Utopia*. New York: Basic Books.

Nyhan, Brendan, Jason Reifler, Sean Richey, and Gary L. Freed. 2014. "Effective Messages in Vaccine Promotion." *Pediatrics* 133(4): e835–42.

Olsaretti, Serena. 2013. "Children and Public Goods." *Philosophy and Public Affairs* 41(3): 226–58.

Pivodic, L., L. Van den Block, K. Pardon, G. Miccinesi, T. Vega Alonso, N. Boffin, G. A. Donker, M. Cancian, A. Lopez-Maside, B. D. Onwuteaka-Philipsen, L. Deliens; EURO IMPACT. 2014. "Burden on Family Carers and Care-Related Financial Strain at the End of Life: A Cross-National Population-Based Study." *European Journal of Public Health* 24(5): 819–26.

Ramsey, Paul. 1976. "The Enforcement of Morals: Nontherapeutic Research on Children." *Hastings Center Report* 6(4): 21–30.

Rawls, John. 1971. *A Theory of Justice.* Cambridge, MA: Harvard University Press.

Reinhard, Susan C., Barbara Given, Nirvana H. Petlick, and Ann Bemis. 2008. "Supporting Family Caregivers in Providing Care." pp. 1–64. In *Patient Safety and Quality: An Evidence-Based Handbook for Nurses,* ed. Ronda Hughes. Rockville, MD: Agency for Healthcare Research and Quality.

Stern, Alexandra, and Howard Markel. 2005. "The History of Vaccines and Immunizations: Familiar Patterns, New Challenges." *Health Affairs* 24(3): 611–21.

Zehr, Howard. 2014. *The Little Book of Restorative Justice.* New York Good Books.

Young Caregivers

GIDEON CALDER

Lula is twelve and the elder of two sisters. She is doing unspectacularly at school, but well enough not to attract special attention. She has an averagely fractious relationship with Ava, her seven-year-old sister. Often they will bicker, of course, and needle or embarrass each other. But beneath all that, and whenever there is trouble, they have a solid, secure bond. Their mother, Katy, is a single parent. For some years, she has been battling mental health problems. This has led to sustained alcohol misuse. Recently she lost her part-time job. She has found herself in a spiral of anxiety and low self-esteem, to which bouts of very heavy drinking have become the stock response. She has good "straight" days where she presents a normal self to the world, but many others are lost to incapacity. For some days every few weeks or so, she is unable to get out of bed.

As time has passed, Lula has effectively taken on the role of Katy's caregiver. At first this was sporadic, only at times of crisis, but it has become normalized. A gradual transfer of responsibilities has taken place: Lula has come to take on the bulk of cooking, cleaning, shopping, and making sure Ava is ready for school. She tries too to persuade her mother to seek help, at least to see a doctor. But for Katy, long proud of her self-sufficiency, this would seem like the ultimate humiliation: a defeat. She feels awkward about what Lula does for her but knows too that she would be drastically adrift without it. Meanwhile, Lula's roles as caregiver and proxy parent are taking up a steadily larger proportion of her life. Yet she doesn't share this, and nobody—relatives, school, nor social services—is aware of the true nature of this domestic setup. In ways that others cannot see it, Lula has come to be highly skilled at coping.

Here we meet the figure of the young caregiver, defined as a five- to seventeen-year-old providing regular unpaid care to a family member who is physically or mentally ill, disabled, experiencing problems related to old age, or misusing drugs or alcohol. The numbers in this category are widely perceived to be rising. In the UK, they are now tracked in official statistics. The 2011 census identified 177,918 young caregivers in the UK, 54% girls and 46% boys (Office for National Statistics 2011; 2013). As elsewhere, this figure is rising, up from 149,929 in 2001. Young caregivers constituted 2.1% of all children in their age group, up from 1.7% in the previous census. While their average age was twelve, the number aged five to seven had risen by 83% since 2001.

This has provoked a kind of moral panic, but not of the conventional sort. Rather than as threats to social order, children in Lula's position are regarded as tragic victims of circumstance—"robbed of childhood," as a typical newspaper headline portrays their "heart-rending plight" (Clark 2007). If there are goods of childhood and goods of parenting, on the familiar understandings these play out consecutively rather than concurrently or alternately. Lula's situation seems to involve an interruption and short-circuiting of the goods of childhood—play, hanging out, self-creation and discovery, a distinctive version of agency—via "parentification." And by arriving at adult responsibilities too soon, she may seem to be missing out too on the goods of parenting. As well as childhood, she may be seen as being "robbed" of key aspects of what makes parenting rewarding. Her position seems out of sync.

Yet such assumptions may be put in question by Lula's own attitude toward her circumstances. Though originally unchosen, she accepts them and has shaped the domestic routines according to her judgments about how things will run best. She does not regard herself as a victim, nor does she seek pity. Indeed, it is vital to her sense of the integrity of her life that she maintains control at home, and her role as a coper. It is a source both of rewards and of a developing sense of her own identity. This is not unusual. Often, people will value family autonomy even when it seems, from the outside, to be giving them a hard deal. We may place a high priority on the scope to make decisions about those closest, even—or perhaps especially—when this imposes heavy burdens on us. Such burdens may feel like blessings, in the context of family bonds. Even if not, they are willingly undertaken.

Thus many unpaid, undersupported young caregivers would like to stay caregivers, even if the costs are high. They may not seek respite. Given the choice, they would prefer that such responsibilities were kept within the family. The costs of intervention from outside would feel to them greater than any imposed by the status quo. Amid the unobtrusive everyday rhythm of their care work, managing well enough, there is "often little likelihood that they will come to the attention of anyone outside their social circle" (McLeod 2012, 64). To deny family autonomy in such cases may seem an affront to justice. We associate such family autonomy most readily with parents steering the lives of their children: making choices about what language they speak, how they will be educated, whether they will be led into religious belief, and so on. But sometimes it applies equally well to the role of a child with regard to a parent, or to another child. If family autonomy suggests a kind of boundary wall around the domestic sphere, Lula is exercising a good deal of agency and time toward maintaining that wall and protecting the status quo. This allows her to fulfill the caring role as she would like it. Nor does she see herself as unfairly lumbered, or a victim in need of rescue.

Still, Lula's well-being is starting to fray. She feels tired more of the time. Friends have noticed that she is often distracted, and sometimes jumpy. She feels separate, detached (O'Dell et al., 2010; Cass, 2007). Though competent at school, her grades are beginning to slip. Because she is not a known caregiver, her role is given no leeway or recognition or credit, beyond Ava—who does not fully appreciate its exceptional nature—and Katy, who is often preoccupied with her own ups and downs. She has no chances to connect with others in a similar position (Clarke and O'Dell 2014, 78). Caring responsibilities seem to be taking up more and more of her available energy, and her general health is dipping. These different factors seem mutually reinforcing. Overlaid, they are having an increasingly weighty impact on the direction of Lula's life. Her situation is quite typical as Figure 5.1 indicates.

We might expect regular care provision to have implications for the health of the caregiver. Results from the 2011 census indicate that those impacts are detrimental. The percentage of people with "Not Good" general health was generally higher among those providing unpaid care compared with those not providing it, and this percentage rose with greater amounts of unpaid care provided. Young caregivers providing upwards of fifty hours of care per week were up to five times more likely to report their general health as being "Not Good."

There are distinctive features of Lula's relationship to Katy and to Ava which reflect customary assumptions about the particular value of familial relationships. Each benefits, in different ways, from their domestic setup and has an interest in sustaining it. Yet each also loses from the very fact that this is their family environment, and that it is a *family* environment. For Lula, as we know, it is taking its toll. Ava too is being accelerated through childhood by the need to deal by herself

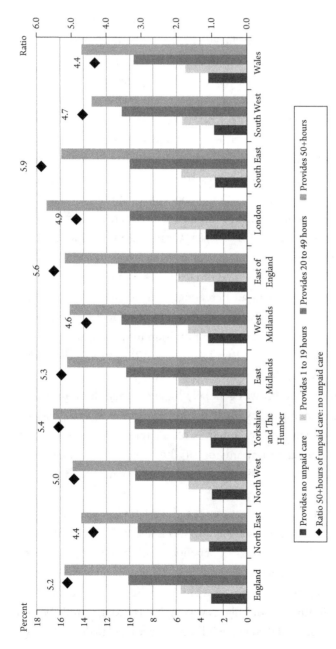

Figure 5.1 Percentage of young unpaid carers with 'Not Good' general health, England and Wales, 2011.

Legend:
- Provides no unpaid care
- Provides 1 to 19 hours
- Provides 20 to 49 hours
- Provides 50+hours
- Ratio 50+hours of unpaid care: no unpaid care

with obstacles of life which her mother might otherwise be helping her around. And Katy is becoming a prisoner of shrinking horizons, dependent in a way which a woman in her forties is not "supposed to be"—let alone in the care of her own pre-teenage child.

This case is emblematic of wider questions of distributive justice: the sharing of resources and caring responsibilities in society, and the impact of this on the life chances of children (and indeed their parents). To what extent, for example, should the situations of Lula and Katy be regarded as the responsibility of outside agencies, and if those agencies intervene, how should they do this, and with what ends in view? It also raises questions about the agency of caregivers, and the extent to which family members have the right to take on roles even when this is detrimental to their well-being. Lula, after all, values and is strongly attached to the very role that may also, from another angle, be seen as thwarting her own further opportunities in life. And it raises questions too about the place of care receivers, in a climate—most starkly in countries such as the UK, where an "austerity" agenda has pared back social budgets—in which funding for social care is waning. For many commentators it is on the brink of collapse (Mortimer 2016). With horizons as they are, the work of family caregivers seems likely only to grow. From the point of view of social justice, young caregivers occupy a distinct and under-analyzed place in that landscape.

REFERENCES

Cass, Bettina. 2007. "Exploring Social Care: Applying a New Construct to Young Carers and Grandparent Carers." *Australian Journal of Social Issues* 42(2): 241–54.

Clark, Laura. 2007. "Thousands of Young Carers Being Robbed of Childhood." *Daily Mail*, May 10, 2007. http://www.dailymail.co.uk/news/article-453794/

Thousands-young-carers-robbed-childhood.html, accessed September 17, 2016.

Clarke, Harriet, and Lindsay O'Dell. 2014. "Disabled Parents and Normative Family Life: The Obscuring of the Lived Experiences of Parents and Children Within Policy and Research Accounts." In *Family Troubles? Exploring Changes and Challenges in the Family Lives of Children and Young People*, ed. J. Ribbens-McCarthy, C. Hooper, and V. Gillies, 75–84. Bristol, UK: Policy Press.

McLeod, Alison. 2012. "What Research Findings Tell Social Workers about Family Support." Unpublished.

Mortimer, Clare. 2016. "UK on Brink of 'Social Care Crisis,' Government Warned." http://www.independent.co.uk/news/uk/politics/social-care-crisis-government-cuts-austerity-elderly-ageing-population-nhs-a7441836.html

O'Dell, Lindsay, Sarah Crafter, Guida Abreu, and Tony Cline. 2010. "Constructing 'Normal Childhoods': Young People Talk About Young Carers." *Disability & Society* 25(6): 643–55.

Office for National Statistics. 2011. *2011 Census*. http://www.ons.gov.uk/census/2011census, accessed September 17, 2016.

Office for National Statistics. 2013. *Providing Unpaid Care May Have an Adverse Effect on Young Carers' General Health*. http://webarchive.nationalarchives.gov.uk/20160105160709/http://www.ons.gov.uk/ons/rel/census/2011-census-analysis/provision-of-unpaid-care-in-england-and-wales--2011/sty-unpaid-care.html, accessed September 17, 2016.

Autism, Family Life, and Epistemic Injustice

RICHARD ASHCROFT

Here is a child. He is cheerful, energetic, lively. He doesn't seem to speak much, but he's a boy, his parents speak two languages to him, he's an only child.

He has been going to nursery since he was about eighteen months old, first for a day a week, then every day. He seemed to hate it at first; separation anxiety? Maybe it's just this nursery. It's a bit industrial. So he goes to a different nursery and all seems fine. He seems to like to play with the same toy, over and over, every day, but he eats and sleeps . . . just like all the other children. One day there's new nursery assistant, who casually says to one of his parents at the end of the day, "He doesn't talk much, does he?" Not ". . . just like all the other children."

At friends for Sunday lunch, one of the hosts says, "Oh, he's talking!" As if this is news. But what is he saying? He's counting the stairs. On their way to the park, he likes to go to all the houses and say the house number. On the way back, he likes to say the numbers of the car-parking spaces, painted onto the road. One of his parents starts to think, "That's a bit autistic, isn't it?" The other dismisses it.

But then, at one of the long series of routine appointments mandated by the NHS to oversee early child development, the health visitor can't engage him in any of her tests. She refers him to a pediatrician. Months later, a speech and language therapist visits the family. She observes him, talks to his parents. She doesn't seem keen to answer any of their questions.

A couple of weeks later, she comes back. The same things happen. She explains that she's not there to diagnose, simply to collect information for the pediatrician. But she's not there to provide reassurance either.

One of the parents spends a lot of time around health researchers, knows about screening tests and false positives, and about the social construction of knowledge and the invention of normality and pathology. There's nothing wrong with this boy; there's a lot wrong with the social processes in play around him. The other parent starts reading up about autism.

Then the appointment with the pediatrician takes place. After an hour of observation and questions: your son has autism spectrum disorder. Here are some leaflets. Here are some numbers to call if you have further questions. This is the clinic you have to attend.

This is my story. Or rather, it is not my story—it's my son's story, his mother's story, the professionals' story, and my story. But I am the one telling it here. These are my recollections of what happened, and I've tried to objectify them by putting them into the third person and confusing who said what and when, but these are the standard ways to control the record of what actually happened, and they fool no one. That's one instance of epistemic injustice to begin with. Do I have the right to tell this story? Maybe; it's my life, after all. But it's not only my life. My son might read this one day. So might his mum. You are already reading it and making up your mind about a few things. There is power in telling a story, in shaping and controlling it, in choosing the language, in deciding what to put in and leave out. But it's a weak sort of power: the meaning of the story is not in my hands, once I've given it to you. Poor me. But power nonetheless.

These other people I am speaking of have no say or control here. The only thing that protects them is my wish to do the right thing, to be honorable. That's a fragile kind of protection. I'm an imperfect judge of my own weaknesses, blind spots, evasions, pride, and self-love. And even if I were a good judge of those things, my attempts at doing the right thing might fail. Human actions so often miss their mark. And you might judge them differently from me.

Perhaps I should not tell my story. Perhaps that is the honorable course. But then I would be passing over in silence the single most important thing about my life: my son, his life, my care and responsibility for him. As a man in philosophy, as in a man in bioethics in particular, the usual path is silence, objectivity, neutrality. Reason. Universals, generalities. No bias, no commitment. The view from nowhere. Yet, as generations of feminist philosophers have taught us, this is to commit injustice. It is to silence those who would speak of life itself; and it is to denigrate and dismiss most of the things that make life itself possible. Care, the flesh, everyday life. *You* shall not speak; and even if you do, what you speak of is *not worth talking about.* Not worth knowing. So taking this attitude commits an epistemic injustice against those who would speak but are silenced, and whose experience is dismissed. And making it normative for the practice of philosophy puts epistemic injustice at the heart of philosophy itself.

I think I should tell my story. But I notice something else: I *can* do so. It's not much of a risk for me. I'm a man (a white man, an able-bodied man, and so much else besides). I acknowledge the responsibility to refuse to continue the epistemic injustice of denying the salience of my daily life—and others'—in my work and in theirs. Yet whereas others (women in philosophy, for instance) risk being considered unreliable or overly emotional or a bad colleague or all the other things people structurally required, forced, to take up caring responsibilities which clash with the requirements of academic and professional life, I have it relatively easy. Just by doing all the things *required* of women who are mothers, I get merit badges for being "sensitive," "thoughtful," "a good dad." We stand here, living our lives, caring for our children and elderly and vulnerable, and all the while the world is handing out scorecards, in a game that is rigged against at least half the participants. There's an epistemic injustice here too: judgment—knowledge—comes unbidden here. Things are known about us, whether or not we want them to be known. *Even when there is nothing to know,* people know it. You do not know whether I am "a good dad"; there is no object of knowledge there, there is nothing to know. But the social fact comes into being, goes around, acquires weight and durability. Independent of the content of that fact (the view that I am or am not a good dad), this unbidden knowledge coalesces and shapes our interactions. Sometimes justice requires not only that we suspend judgment, but that we make no judgment at all, leave room for there to be no judgment.

I could, therefore, not tell my story. There are lots of others to tell stories of autism and family life, and when our son was first diagnosed I read a lot of them. I wanted to know what to expect; I wanted ideas of what to do; I wanted hope. But I suppose most of all I wanted other stories than the ones which were already in control of our lives at that point. One thing I had not realized before I became a father is that parenthood involves continual comparison. You watch other children and think, "Does mine do that?" Others watch yours, too. I spent a lot of time wondering why my son wouldn't do some things that other children, even children younger than him, could do, and being proud when he could do things that other children could not. I fought hard against my tendencies to be the stereotypical middle-class competitive parent, but worry and joy are inherent to being a parent and sometime these are things I worried or was joyful about.

Nonetheless, the story of your child is not made only by you—or by the child. Other stories circulate, and sometimes they are the ones in control. The NHS is a wonderful institution and really comes into its own in supporting families through pregnancy and into early child-hood. It does this through statistics and the mobilization of profession-als trained to collate, analyze, assess, and judge on the basis of those. One inevitable consequence of this is that they—and we—come to be obsessed with charts and graphs, deviations from the norm. Your child cannot do this, this, and this, and so there is a problem. And I fought with that: Where do your statistics come from? How did you decide these were the criteria? What's so great about normal? And later on, where is the evidence that this intervention is effective and safe? On the one hand, their statistics; on the other, our lovely boy, so happy, so delightful. The only child we have, the child who came late and unex-pectedly, and the only child we had any close day-to-day contact with. One narrative of science and professional judgment came into contact with another narrative of personal daily lived experience.

So much of the literature around autism focuses on this personal daily lived experience, and various conflicts of epistemic author-ity. Each family, and each individual, arrives at their own unstable accommodation with the different knowledges in play: the statisti-cal, developmental, neuroscientific, professional, institutional, social, autobiographical . . . From the nursery school teacher who "knew" that something was different about our son simply from having spent a lot of time with small children, to the relative who "knew" that an autism diagnosis was not a tragedy because "they all have a special talent, don't they?" to the health visitor who didn't know much other than "this child meets the criteria for a referral" and the speech thera-pist who "knew" our son was autistic but also "knew" that she was not allowed to tell us. I don't put "knew" in scare quotes here to sug-gest that they were wrong or even that there is no fact of the matter, but rather to emphasize that these were the appropriate knowledges for these people in these places in the structure and process of pro-ducing our lives out of the raw material of daily existence. Relative to these positions in that structure and process these knowledges could be mistaken, but they were and are authoritative. They have power, and they are hard to resist.

In time one becomes inculcated into new knowledges and it's less a question of resistance than of learning how to use and shape these knowledges, build alliances, and add one's own stories to the polyphony (cacophony?) of narratives. But at the moment I described at the outset my experience was of something else: epistemic catastrophe. I had thought I knew certain things about my son; I was utterly wrong. I thought I knew some things about his future; I was utterly deluded. I thought I knew something about my own intelligence and ability to process critical information and ideas and theories; I was a perfect fool. Everyone else around me knew things about my son; I knew nothing. It is possible, it turns out, to be epistemically unjust to oneself—to mislead oneself about one's own life by pretending to knowledge which is utterly mistaken and self-serving. But also to misunderstand that this too shall pass and that one is not an absolute idiot and that sometimes events, beyond knowledge, actual material-practical-existential events, can change your life.

A final epistemic injustice. I have given my son no voice here. He can speak for himself, and he does. The stories around autism that are in play in the mainstream of our culture are now multiple and various and relatively high profile. Yet we still relatively rarely hear from autistic people about their lives, experiences, desires, hopes, fears, needs. It's not that they don't articulate them; though many autistic people have communication impairments, many are quite able to speak for themselves and do. But we don't listen, we don't enable them, we don't make space for them. To deny ourselves this knowledge is epistemic injustice to them and to ourselves; to deny that they have knowledge, even if sometimes they know differently, is also epistemic injustice. But I am not the one to make this argument: I invite you to leave this space open for autistic people to tell their own stories, as they want them to be told.

INDEX

aging, 89, 90, 91
autism, 155–56
autonomy, 47–48, 115–16, 123–24, 126–28, 130–31, 159–60, 168–72

Baier, Annette, 8–9, 19

cancer, 70–72, 73, 77–78
care. *See* family; healthcare; nursing home/residential; social care/home care
care workers/domestic workers, 89
family caregivers, 4–5, 19–20, 26–28, 98, 112–13, 115, 116–17, 155, 164, 166–69
feminist approaches to, 50–51
pressure of care, 26–28
Carsten, Janet, 2–3, 53–54
children/childhood. *See* family
abuse, 157
as carers, 155
immunization, 169–72
rights and interests, 56–58, 158–59

disability, 27–28, 50–51, 59–60
disclosure, 37–45
donor conception, 16

ethics, 6, 25–26, 27–28, 33, 131–33, 161–62
See also healthcare ethics

family. *See* care; genetics
biology of, 28–34, 75–76, 93–94
change, 2–3, 4–5
children, 19–20, 29, 37–38, 43–44, 62–63, 89, 162, 186–87
cultural norms, 2–3, 89
harm, 18, 21, 22–24, 51–52, 157
identity, 19–23, 24–25, 28, 33–34, 43, 49, 51–52, 53–55, 60–61, 75, 94–95, 96
importance of, chapter one, 48–50
narratives of, 6–7, 19–22, 38–39, 53–55, 60–64
obligation, 76–77, 91, 113–14, 128–30
of origin, 20–21, 51–52
responsibilities to care, 1–2, 4–6, 7, 17, 19–20, 23–28, 90–91, 92–93, 94, 95–97, 98–99, 112–14, 116–17, 121, 163–66
same-sex, 6–7, 16
siblings, 147–53
sociology of, 2–3, 61–64
stress, 26–28
varied forms of, 7–8, 17, 47–48, 51–52, 61–64, 72–75

feminist perspectives, 25–26, 47–48, 50–51, 104, 150, 185

gender. *See* parenthood
  care responsibilities, 24–25, 89, 97, 98, 150–51, 162–63, 164
  change, 4–5
genetics, 38–39, 47–48

Hardwig, John, 51–52
healthcare. *See* patient/s
  consent, 28–29, 59–60, 96–97, 151, 171
  counseling, 38, 42, 44, 139–44
  decision-making, 77–78, 118–19, 168–72
    shared decision-making, 1–2, 119–26, 134–35
  healthcare ethics, 25–26, 27–28
  home-based healthcare, 24, 109–12, 138–39, 140–44, 163–64
  hospital, 2, 25, 26, 89
  innovations, 4, 18
  practitioners/professionals, 121, 134–35
  role of family, chapter four, 1–2, 19–20, 27–28, 47–49, 60–61, 139–44, 163
Ho, Anita, 60–61
home, 26, 99, 172–73, 178

identity. *See* family; narrative
  relational, 50–51, 57–59, 60–61
illness, 48–49, 163–64, 166, 171
  chronic illness, 7–8, 10, 21–22, 24–25, 118
  serious/acute illness, 23, 26
inequality, 5, 62–64

justice, chapter five, 8–9, 97–98, 178–79, 181, 184–86, 188

Levine, Carol, 1–2
Lindemann, Hilde/Nelson, Hilde
  Lindemann, 1, 6–7, 8–9, 21, 27–28, 30, 48–50, 52, 100–1

moral/morality, 2–3, 7–9, 17–18, 21, 27–28, 76–78, 84–85, 159–60, 161
  judgements, 2–3, 22
  naturalized moral epistemology, 8–9
  responsibility, 28–34, 77–78, 84–85, 90–91, 92–99, 123–24, 126–29, 168–69

narrative, 6–7, 53–55, 81, 82, 86–87, 186–87, 188
  See also family
Nelson, James Lindemann, 1, 27–28, 30, 48–50, 55, 100–1
nursing home, 89–90

O'Neill, Onora, 56–58
organ donation, 118–19, 127–28

parents, 16, 56–57, 59–60, 84–85, 97, 98, 118, 162, 164, 169–72, 176–78, 186
  gender of, 89, 164–65
  responsibilities of, 56–60, 158–59
  responsibilities for, 89
patient/s, chapter four, 1–2, 16–17, 18, 24–25, 27–28, 43–45, 48–49, 106–7, 159, 168–69

relationality, 36–37, 40–42, 43–44, 47–48, 50–55, 57–61, 66, 115, 118–21, 123–26, 129–31, 133, 134–35
responsibility. *See* family; gender; moral/ morality; parents
rights, 56–58, 101–2, 104

social care/home care, 1–6, 50, 54–55, 89, 181

Verkerk, Marian, 32
vulnerability, 32, 51–52, 55–60, 92, 97

Walker, Margaret Urban, 32, 92–93, 97
welfare state, 90–91